To Dave & Phyl[illegible]

There's always an angle –
I send this to you with very
best wishes, knowing that you
will send me yours, and
I'll wind up ahead.

Thanks for your
support while I was
writing this.

Budd

22 May, 1975

Health Care for Migrant Workers: Policies & Politics

Health Care for Migrant Workers: Policies & Politics

Budd N. Shenkin, M.D., M.A.P.A.

Ballinger Publishing Company • Cambridge, Mass.
A Subsidiary of J.B. Lippincott Company

International Standard Book Number: 0-88410-108-8

Library of Congress Catalog Card Number: 74-13911

Printed in the United States of America

Library of Congress Cataloging in Publication Data

Shenkin, Budd N

Health care for migrant workers: policies and politics.

Includes bibliographical references.

1. Migrant agricultural laborers–Medical care–United States. 2. Rural health services–United States. I. Title. [DNLM: 1. Delivery of health care–U.S. 2. Rural health–U.S. 3. Transients and migrants. WA390 S546h].

RA448.5.M5S52 362.8'5 74-13911

ISBN 0-88410-108-8

Table of Contents

List of Tables

List of Figures

Preface

I started writing this book in the spring of 1970 as my nearly two year stint as an administrator of the Migrant Health Program in Washington, D.C. was coming to an end. By that time, my bureaucratic allies and I had made some significant policy breakthroughs with the MHP; I wanted to solidify and possibly advance those gains by getting our basic reasoning down on paper. Paper, I had learned, has a way of living in the bureaucracy and surviving the departure of individuals.

I had first got involved with the MHP by accident in 1968 when, in common with many other young physicians graduating from internships, I signed up with the Public Health Service as an alternative to the draft. My interest in government and politics led me to the Division of Medical Care Administration, which soon became the Community Health Service. A series of subsequent events largely beyond my control conspired to assign me to the MHP.

Even though the assignment occurred through happenstance, it was an accident for which I was prepared. I found the clear-cut mission to serve the exploited particularly seductive in contrast to the less partisan attitudes taken by many other programs. As I administered the program, it soon became clear that its policies had grave deficiencies. Other newcomers to the MHP felt the same way, and in short order two factions developed, one composed of the MHP "old guard" opposing change, and one composed of newcomers who wanted to "modernize" the MHP policies, essentially as is advocated in this book. Our faction waged a hard, bureaucratic fight for what we thought were right, justice, and the American way. At the end, we could show for our efforts about seven comprehensive, consumer-based projects with about $500,000 yearly budgets, and a set of (unapproved) project guidelines, later modified to become official MHP regulations.

As the new projects were being funded, it was clear that our victories could well be temporary, and that momentum for change was rapidly vanishing.

A way to assure continuing influence seemed to be through the written word. So I tried to compose a policy analysis of the MHP that would (1) convince policymakers in the Administration and Congress that the new style comprehensive projects were rational and desirable, (2) give ammunition to other advocates of this policy, and (3) at the very least, direct future policy considerations to the questions we were concerned with. Even though it has taken longer than I foresaw to complete that analysis, the primary purpose has remained the same.

I thought initially that the analysis would be rather easy to do, but as I kept trying, it became harder and harder. Many of the assumptions we had relied on had to be challenged, and I didn't know how to deal with the nonascertainable assertions of medical care experts that were really no more than opinions. Although I had a good feel for the politics and administration of migrant health, I found it difficult to deal with them explicitly. Most importantly, I was so deeply involved emotionally that everything I wrote came out as the self-righteous denunciations of an impassioned young man. So, I wrote down what I could and kept it in reserve for awhile.

Fortunately, I had chosen to spend the next year taking my master's degree at the Graduate School of Public Policy at Berkeley. Through the year the faculty strengthened my conviction that an effective policy study should not only analyze the issue in question, but also the administrative and political conditions that have to be met by a proposed policy. Emotion ebbing and theoretical knowledge increasing, I saw how I might write a convincing policy study using interdisciplinary techniques. Since the faculty could not supply me with a model analysis to learn from, I added a second purpose to my writing agenda: to produce a model policy analysis incorporating administrative and political analyses.

I wrote the bulk of the semi-final draft during the next academic year (1971–72), which I spent as a visiting researcher at the Economic Research Institute at the Stockholm School of Economics. As I wrote, it occurred to me that two other, smaller purposes might be served. First, many of the factors that are peculiar to low-salience programs are nicely illustrated by considering this case—for instance, the importance that one or two individuals at a relatively low level can assume, and the systematic trading-off that sacrifices these smaller issues for larger ones. Second, many may be interested in, and even find research guidance from, the problems I encounter with gaps in medical care knowledge that often leave arguments perched precariously on unproved assumptions. For instance, it seems absurd that we have no notion of the various cost-effectiveness ratios of medical procedures, which could be used to guide administrators with a paucity of resources. We also have very little hard information to guide us in allocating money to environmental and medical efforts.

APPROACH

The practically-oriented primary purpose of the book dictated a comprehensive approach. It was not enough to analyze the root causes of ill health among migrants and to find policies that would theoretically improve the MHP; a better policy would have to be consonant with the current administrative capabilities of HEW, or at least necessary administrative improvements would have to be feasible. Likewise, the political atmosphere would have to be analyzed to find if recommended policies were feasible or not, and to identify specific ways to gain acceptance of the policies.

Choosing to be comprehensive carries a latent implication of not delving too deeply into any one aspect. I have had to accept that trade-off, and have therefore had to rely on work done by others, or assumptions, or have had to stop my reasoning at unsatisfactory spots. The comprehensive approach does have the virtue, however, of enabling would-be researchers to select a subject with an eye to possible policy results. I hope this book does stimulate some such work. Many policy areas, in fact, could use such comprehensive studies to direct further research efforts, which are currently all too often chosen haphazardly.

Despite its comprehensiveness, this study is nonetheless incremental in philosophy. It analyzes the problem from first principles, but then seeks to find the best feasible next step, starting with the program, policy, and other conditions that now exist. It is even conservative in its incrementalism, assuming no great power shifts, but only the influence of the forces now in existence. I wish I could do more. It is far from satisfying to assume no change in working conditions, no improvement in unionization, no increase in political-economic power, and to project no new programs ensuring minimum annual income, or comprehensive housing for agricultural workers. I only hope that by being so conservative I have not contributed to a self-fulfilling prophesy.

HOW TO READ THIS BOOK

I doubt that many people will want to read this book straight through–in fact, no matter what your purpose, I recommend that you don't. The book's organization facilitates the reader's getting a quick overview of the arguments, and picking and choosing which areas to examine more closely. Each chapter is summarized at the end, and I suggest reading these five summaries *seriatim* as an introduction. Each section within the chapters is generally also summarized; I suggest proceeding next to that level, and then finally to the basic narrative if you want.

Although the constant summarizing gets a bit repetitious, I thought it was necessary to accommodate readers who might be looking for quite different things.

Foreword

The past decade has seen great progress in our understanding of medical care systems. We know much more than we previously did about our public policy choices in organizing and financing medical care for the general population, and for various needy subgroups as well. In the Congress we have been trying to make sure that our programs keep pace with that knowledge, and that they constantly review their progress and problems and upgrade themselves. While the federal administrators themselves have done a commendable job, voluntary groups and private citizens with special interests in these programs have made important contributions to help the government serve the people as best it can.

In this context, Dr. Shenkin has written an important book. The Migrant Health Program can be a strong asset to these harvesters of the fields, and when my aide Brian Biles and I became aware of Dr. Shenkin's work, we were convinced that services could be greatly improved if we were to utilize many of his ideas. I am hopeful that the new Migrant Health Law of 1974, which incorporates many of his ideas, will in fact serve migrant workers with higher quality services provided more efficiently than was formerly the case.

Dr. Shenkin's book is important in another way. It serves as a fine example of how a physician can use the newer tools of social science to derive a policy that is able to be implemented in light of political realities. Too often have plans for health care been put foreward without any chance of enactment because the author forgot to assign dollar figures to his plans, or neglected to consider the forces extant in the political arena. This book should guide those who want their thoughts and deliberations to make a practical difference in the foreseeable future.

William R. Roy, M.D.

List of Abbreviations

APHA	American Public Health Association
ASPE	Assistant Secretary for Planning and Evaluation (Department of Health, Education, and Welfare)
AWHMA	Agricultural Workers Health and Medical Association
CHMTA	Comprehensive Health Manpower Training Act
CHS	Community Health Service
DMCA	Division of Medical Care Administration
DOL	Department of Labor
EPA	Environmental Protection Agency
FSA	Farm Security Agency
HSMHA	Health Services and Mental Health Administration
MHP	Migrant Health Program
MHPRC	Migrant Health Project Review Committee
MLAP	Migrant Legal Action Program
NHC	Neighborhood Health Center
NHSC	National Health Service Corps
NLRA	National Labor Relations Act
NTA	Nurse Training Act
OMB	Office of Management and Budget
OMICA	Organized Migrants in Community Action
OSHA	Occupational Safety and Health Act
UFW	United Farm Workers
USDA	United States Department of Agriculture

Health Care for Migrant Workers: Policies & Politics

Chapter One

The Problem of Migrant Health

Migrant agricultural workers have been needed for the last one hundred years in America because we have chosen from that time and even earlier to have very large farms rather than family farms, to have these farms specialize rather than diversify the crops and consequently the time and intensity of labor need, and to mechanize extensively those processes amenable to machine operations.[1] Ownership of the land in California is so concentrated, for instance, that "3.7 million acres of California farmland are owned by 45 corporate farms. Thus, nearly half of the agricultural land in the state, and probably three-quarters of the prime irrigated land, is owned by a tiny fraction of the population."[2] The origin of this pattern arises from the size of the original land grants made in the southern states, the failure of the government to break up the large Spanish and Mexican land grants in the Southwest and California when those areas were annexed into the United States (and later), and the corruption of such laws that were made to foster homesteading.[3] Today, the owners of agribusiness and thus the employers of migrants, are increasingly large diversified companies and banks with interlocking directorates.[4] Whether or not such large holdings are economically more profitable than smaller holdings is not clear: governmental granting, pricing, and taxing policies, and the oligopsonistic advantages of bigness obscure that question.[5] The social effect on the countryside and its populace is more clear: where large land holdings dominate, this is no small, integrated rural community life of towns, schools, and farms traditionally considered the basis of the American value system, such as has been found in the past in New England and parts of the Midwest.

Migrant workers can easily be seen, and have most often been painted, as the most direct victims of our agricultural system. John Steinbeck immortalized one set of them as persons, and Carey McWilliams as victims of a system and a history.[6]

This book, however, does not seek to contribute to the overthrow of the system, however worthwhile that objective might appear, but rather to sub-optimize by determining how best to improve the health of these migrant workers through a federal program that assumes the continuation of that system. The task of this first chapter, then, is to develop a factual analysis of why migrants might need a Migrant Health Program, as has existed since 1962, and what problems such a program must meet. We shall look at the hard facts that describe the migrants' poor state of health, and the way of life that contributes to it. Then we shall look at the system of rural health care in America, that also contributes to the migrants' state of health, and which must be dealt with by any policy the government is to adopt. Finally, we shall combine these facts into a systematic schema of interactions describing the production of poor health among migrants, and consider some of the possibilities for intervention.

If this analytic approach be more boring than the great majority of writings on the deprivations of migrants, at least it cannot be accused of inciting the emotions to unwarranted conclusions.

I DESCRIPTION OF THE MIGRANTS

Statistics on migrants are easy to come by, but accurate ones are not. Migrant statistics are generated in the federal government mostly by the Departments of Labor (DOL) and Agriculture (USDA), but they themselves admit that their figures are usually useful only for gross estimates. That statistics on migrants are far from precise and useful for those who want to use migrants rather than serve them, supplies an insight into the migrants' place in America. They are far off the beaten track, and the two government departments that deal with them most do not even know how many there are.

A. General Description

Each year as crops ripen progressively more northward, there is a consequent demand for field laborers along the route. The duration of each job is variable, but the average migrant works in several different locations during the year. In a survey of migrants in Homestead, Florida, 22 percent of Chicano families and 38 percent of blacks went to only one upstream location; 61 percent of Chicanos and 54 percent of blacks went to two or three.[7] Although the wages are poor and the work sporadic and extremely demanding physically, and travel overhead is very high, there is a superabundance of persons willing to do the work. There were in 1971, according to USDA, probably about 172,000 migrant laborers over fourteen years of age in the total seasonal farm worker force of about 2.6 million.[8] The Department of Health, Education and Welfare (HEW) and others estimate the total of migrant persons (including "non-working" family members) at one million.

Definitions of migrancy vary among administrative agencies, but the basic intent of definition is a person who moves so far away from the place he calls home to work in the fields, that he must stay away from home overnight for some period of time. In addition to the domestic farm workers, a large number of foreign nationals, Mexicans, Canadians, British West Indians, and others, swell the ranks of farm workers (see figure 1-1). The Mexican influx, once controlled by the bracero program, now confined to "green card" permanent immigrant and non-"green card" illegals, forces the migrants northward, since they are underbid for jobs in their homebase areas by the Mexicans. Migrants also ply their trade for want of better alternatives; since migrant children get extremely poor schooling, they grow up unable to qualify for many jobs. Other reasons for migrating are tradition, cultural mores among Mexicans and Mexican-Americans that endorse the migrants' hard work as morally laudable, and discrimination against migrants in other occupations.

Migrants work for small and large farms, some going back to the same one repeatedly, more changing from year to year. Despite mechanization that diminishes the demand for agricultural workers, most authorities seem to agree that there will be many migrants for many years to come, even if an effective higher minimum wage should be established.

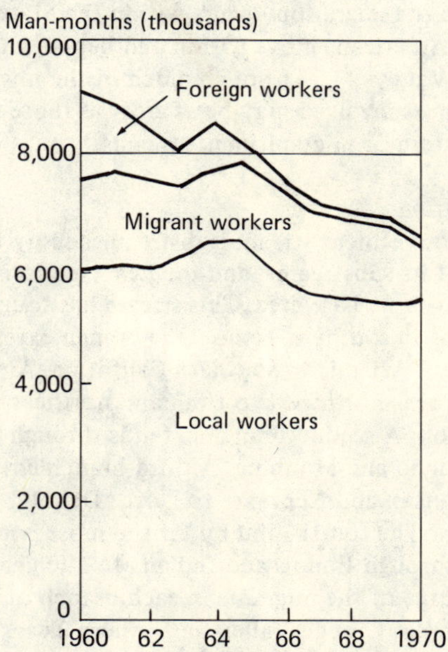

Figure 1-1. Man-Months of Employment of Seasonal Hired Farmworkers by Type of Worker, 1960 to 1970. Source: "Rural Manpower Developments," U.S. Department of Labor, May 1971.

Migrants follow the maturing crops in three general streams. Their travels fall into a coherent, if highly varied, pattern. Figure 1–2 depicts the streams as they existed in 1965. Observe that there are three distinct home base areas from which migrants move northward: southern California, southern Texas, and southern Florida. Note that the stream originating in Texas fans out into the entire midcontinent region and intermingles with the other two streams. Each stream shows a large component of intrastate movement within the home base state . . .

California Stream

The California stream is the most populous and best defined. At the peak of the season, California employs 61,000 migrant workers, about half of whom come from another state. This number represents nearly one-fourth of the total U.S. migratory labor force. California also accounts for one-fourth of the total U.S. annual man-months of migrant worker employment (according to 1968 estimates of the Bureau of Employment Security).

Most migrants in this stream are Mexican-American; however, the Washington and Oregon component of the stream do have a high proportion (40%) of "Anglos."

Most of the migration occurs within the State of California as Mexican-Americans move within and between the San Joaquin and Imperial Valleys . . . Although much of the migration is intrastate, the distances involved may be as great as those traveled by migrants in the eastern or midcontinent streams.

Midcontinent Stream

The midcontinent stream is distinguished by the multitude and dispersion of its substreams, and the heavy concentration of migrants in the Texas home base area. This stream has four basic branches, all originating in southern Texas. One branch extends through New Mexico and Arizona to southern California. A major offshoot of this branch moves northwest to Utah and northeast Nevada and finally to Washington. A second branch extends through Colorado to Washington, Idaho and Montana. A third branch extends through Oklahoma, Kansas, and Nebraska to North Dakota, Minnesota, and Wisconsin. The fourth, and by far the most populous branch, extends through Illinois and Indiana to Michigan and Ohio.

The source of the migrants in each branch of the stream is primarily the lower Rio Grande Valley in southern Texas. There, in Hidalgo County alone, approximately 37,500 migrant workers and their dependents reside. The migrants who reside there, and those who move in the stream itself, are predominantly Mexican-American. There is a small percentage of Indians who also migrate in this stream.

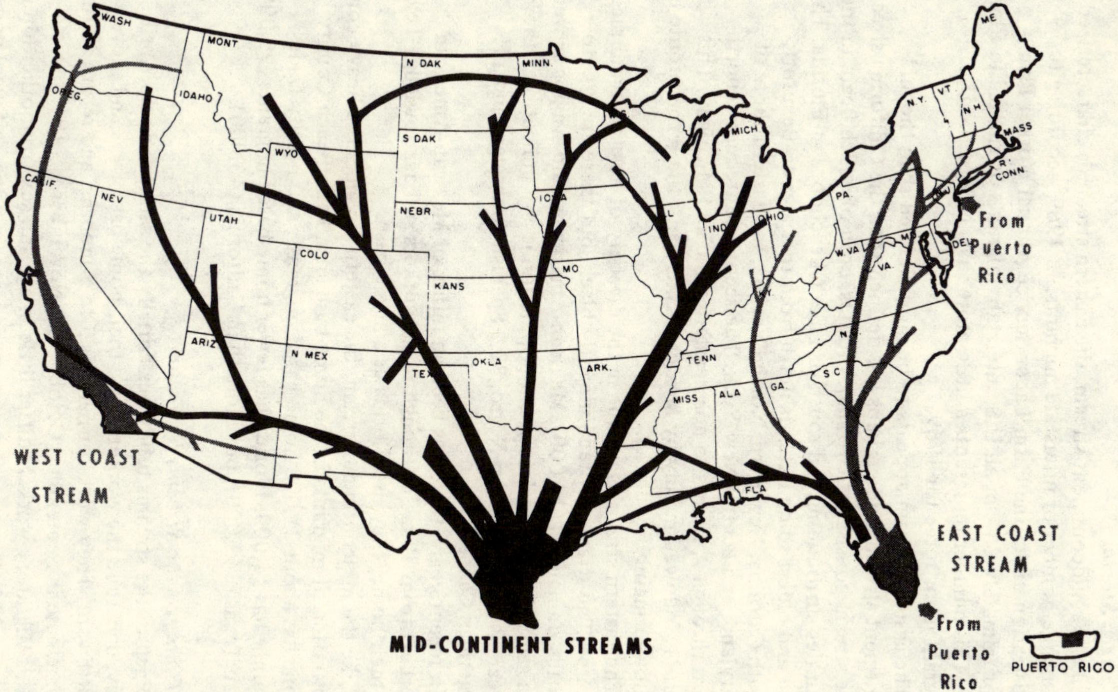

Figure 1–2. Travel Patterns of Seasonal Migratory Agricultural Workers. Note: This map shows the major directions of the northward migratory movement of domestic agricultural workers. The movement is reversed as the crop season ends in the northern states and the workers drift back to their home base areas—for many of them, southern California, Texas and Florida. Source: Public Health Service Publication No. 540, August 1966.

The midcontinent stream is the least well defined of the three major streams, but it probably involves the largest number of *interstate* migrants in the country. . . .

Eastern Stream

Like the midcontinent stream, the eastern stream is characterized by a large number of interstate migrants. In 1969, according to registration under the Farm Labor Service Annual Worker Plan, approximately 26% of all U.S. interstate migrants originated in Florida. This number represents a little more than 10% of the U.S. migrant labor force for 1969.

The eastern stream appears to be more defined than the midcontinent stream, and perhaps less defined than the California stream. The stream consists of two major routes, both of which begin in the counties surrounding and south of Lake Okeechobee in Florida. The first and oldest route extends north from that area to Beaufort, South Carolina; New Bern, North Carolina; the eastern shore of Maryland, and central New York. The second route moves northward through Alabama to northeastern Ohio and Michigan. This route is followed mainly by Mexican-Americans; the former route is followed mainly by blacks.

The eastern stream is unique in the diversity of its ethnic and racial groups. The stream is predominantly black, but there are Puerto Ricans, Jamaicans (14,000), Mexican-Americans, and Anglos as well. If a sample of Florida's migrant population is any indication,[a] the stream is 56% American Negro, 32% Spanish-American, and 11% American Caucasian.

In recent years, there has been an influx of Mexican-American workers from Texas. Although these workers still acknowledge Texas as their home, they use Florida as a home base.

Like the midcontinent stream, the eastern stream has a heavy concentration of migrants in the home base area. Palm Beach County alone has about 21,000 home based migrants, and nearby Dade County has 11,000. Florida has fewer home based migrants (92,000) than Texas (143,000), but more than California (43,000). . . .

Timing of the Streams by Season

Each of the streams follows essentially the same cycle. In April, May, and June the workers leave their home base areas and move northward. They work for perhaps 3 to 5 months, and return to the home base in September, October and November. . . .[9]

. . . Migratory workers differ little in age and sex from other hired farmworkers. They are a young work force; in 1967 half were under 25 years of age. A fourth were teenages 14 through 17 years old. . . .

[a]Dr. John E. Kleinert, Migrant Children in Florida, Phase II Report, p. 76, University of Miami, Florida Migratory Child Survey Center, 1969.

> The migratory farm wage force of 1967 was predominantly male in all age groups. Only one-fourth of the migrants were female.[10]

On the other hand, other studies show a much more nearly equal distribution of males and females.[11] The ethnic composition of the stream is likewise in some dispute, some estimates asserting that 15 percent are black and 25 percent Chicano, others that "most interstate migrant workers are Mexican-Americans, . . . (and) most migrant workers travel interstate as opposed to intrastate,"[12] and yet most intrastate migration takes place in California, where the majority are Mexican-American. Most experts think the majority are Chicanos.

The families tend to be large, Chicanos estimated to have 6.5 family members on the average in Texas. The Homestead survey showed Chicanos with 5.5 members per family, and blacks, 4.9.[13]

> Although some migratory farmwork was done in almost every State, half of the total man-months of migratory worker employment in 1967 occurred in five States: California, Florida, Michigan, Texas, and Washington. . . . In December 1965, 40 % of the migratory workers were living in the geographic region extending from Texas east to the Atlantic Ocean and north through Maryland and Delaware. The remaining workers were about equally distributed in the northern and western regions of the United States.[14] (See figure 1-3).

Community Change, Incorporated, estimated in 1971 that "the vast majority of home-based migrants and their dependents are concentrated in these states: Florida (87,170); Texas (111,267); and California (114,950)."[15] They further found that fifty-nine counties could be described as migrant impact counties with more than 4,000 migrants at some time of the year. Of these, twenty-one were homebase, twenty-one mixed and seventeen upstream. Table 1-1 shows that in the former two types of area the duration of stay was greater than eight months; in the latter, thirteen counties hosted stays of from four to eight months, and four counties less than four months. A more exact breakdown of populations appears in table 1-2. The basic data Community Change, Incorporated, developed appears in Appendix C.

It is often said that migrants are generally indistinguishable from the rural poor around them in the homebase areas. This is probably true. No statistics are available to indicate the facts of the situation, but it is common knowledge in the areas in question that farm workers may choose to migrate in certain years but not in others, there being little difference in their economic status whether they do or not. The upstream areas are different in this respect, however; the migrant workers often live apart from the local resident farm workers, and are subject to more severe conditions. The migrants have special camps, special stores, and often language and racial differences.

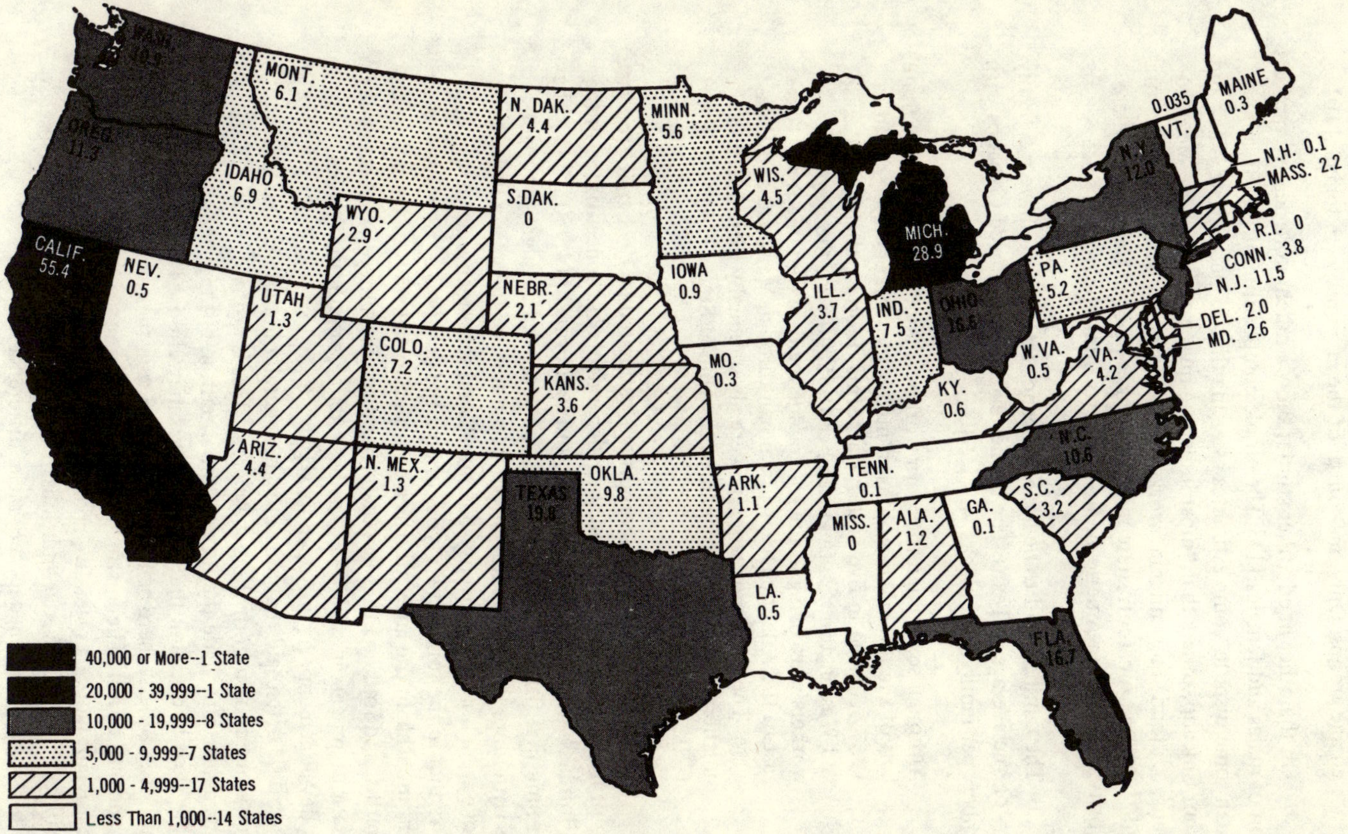

Figure 1-3. Peak Employment of Domestic Migrant Farmworkers, 1970 (In Thousands). Source: "Rural Manpower Developments," U.S. Department of Labor, May 1971.

Table 1-1. Migrant Demography—Length of Stay in Fifty-Nine High-Impact Counties

Duration of Stay	*Location*		
	Home Base	*Mixed*	*Upstream*
0–4 months	–	–	4
4–8 months	–	–	13
8–12 months	21	21	–

Source: Community Change, Inc.

> The income statistics of the migrants are shockingly bad.
>
> One-fourth of all migratory workers were members of families with cash incomes of less than $2,000 in 1965, and the median income of households headed by migratory workers are $2,735 in 1965. Annual family incomes of less than $3,000 were characteristic of nearly three-fifths of household heads and wives who did farm wage-work on the road.[16]
>
> The migrant workers' average annual income was $1,630 for 118 days of farm and non-farm work. From farmwork, migrants averaged $987 and 79 days of employment, while non-farm work provided them an average of $642 and 39 days of employment in 1971.[17]

In 1972 the average migrant worked 141 days and earned $2,179.[18] As if these statistics were not bad enough, one must also remember that migrants can be subject to large expenses for transportation, wage deductions by crew leaders, rents for lodgings, etc.

Almost 90 percent of Chicano heads of household in Homestead have not completed the ninth grade, and this is true of 57 percent of the blacks.[19]

> Every major report on the living and working conditions of migratory workers and their families emphasizes almost without exception the

Table 1-2. Migrant Demography—Number of Migrants in Fifty-Nine High-Impact Counties

Number of Migrants	*Location*			
	Home Base	*Mixed*	*Upstream*	*Total*
4,000–7,999	12	5	11	28
8,000–11,999	6	5	4	15
12,000–23,999	1	9	0	10
24,000–	2	2	2	6
Total	21	21	17	59

Source: Community Change, Inc.

> shocking and immediate necessity for housing improvements. Migrants live in dilapidated, drafty, ramshackle houses that are cold and wet in the winter, and leaky, steaming, and excessively hot in the summer. Insufficient ventilation, poor or no mattresses, unsanitary privies and bathing devices, and unsanitary storage and disposal of garbage and refuse are too often the prevailing conditions.[20]

The Migrant Research Project found in Michigan in 1969 that

> 34% of the units had wet floors, 29% leaking roofs, 25% leaking floors. . . . a clear pattern of violations can be discerned in a myriad of important areas such as drainage; maintenance of an adequate, accessible and safe water supply; and provisions for recreational areas, eating facilities and lighting for common areas and facilities adjacent to the camp. . . . Overcrowding of these basically unsound units further accentuated the deficiencies found. For example, beds were not always available for the inhabitants and, when provided, almost invariably served more than two persons. . . . basic sanitation problems were also documented. For instance, only 22% of the camps provided a toilet for each housing unit. For the remaining units, the common privies provided were found to be insufficient in number and badly maintained and ventilated. The camps were also regarded as hazardous by our observers.[21]

B. State of Health

Valid health statistics of migrants and of the rural poor are hard to find. It is not possible to distinguish the state of health of the migrants from that of the general rural poor, because it is very difficult to get specific data on even the rural poor, and the surveys taken of migrant health conditions have been very limited in scope and technique. The migrant health projects operated under federal grants are subject to limitations, discussed below, that make use of their figures inadvisable.

Despite the limitations of the figures, however, a strong case can be made that the state of health of both the migrants and the rural poor is generally wretched.

In the United States poor people are sicker than non-poor people, blacks and Chicanos are sicker than whites, and rural people are sicker than urban people. The sicker groups generally get less medical care.[22] Since all migrants are poor and rural, and most (we think) are black or Chicano, we would expect the migrants to be among the least well groups of persons in the country, just on the basis of this general data. In addition, the occupation of agricultural worker is the third most hazardous one in the country, after mining and construction. Not only is work on the farm subject to a high accident rate, but the use of pesticides provides a heretofore little recognized additional hazard.

One report estimates that one-sixth of all California farm workers are injured with pesticides each year,[23] another indicates a high degree of chronic pesticide poisoning in farm workers in Colorado.[24]

Some local surveys of migrants give a more specific picture. One migrant health clinic in San Luis Obispo County in California in 1967–68 did diagnostic screening of their migrant patients.[25] They found that 29 to 37 percent of the non-pregnant women tested has anemia, depending on the standard of normality used. Twelve percent of the adult men tested were definitely anemic, and 38 percent of the children tested were definitely anemic. Diabetes mellitus was found by screening blood sugar levels to be probable, but not certain, in 16 percent of the persons screened. Urinary tract abnormalities were found to be present in 14 percent of the adult male patients examined. Skin tests for tuberculosis turned up "an extremely high yield of positive reactors." There was a "high yield" of positive findings for the pap smears taken to detect carcinoma of the cervix. Blood tests taken to detect syphilis, however, detected only an average amount for the California population.

The Colorado Migrant Council in 1969 sponsored a survey of 300 migrant Chicano children less than six years old. The families were generally representative of the Colorado migrant agricultural population.[26] Conversations with parents revealed an infant mortality of 63 per 1,000 live births (compared to the national infant mortality figures for 1969 of 20.7 for all groups, 18.4 for white persons, and 31.6 for all others [27]). Physical and biochemical examinations revealed many signs of malnutrition, including much stunting of growth, anemia, and a 55 percent prevalence of vitamin A deficiency, 20 percent quite severe.

Delgado, Brumback, and Deaver showed in 1961 that the diets of black migrants in Florida were nutritionally deficient.[28] Confirmatory biochemical evidence of nutritional insufficiency was produced by a 1965 study of East Coast black migrants in the New York camp.[29] In fact, in comparing their nutritional status with other groups, "the migrant workers had the lowest average values for five of the seven indices studies: serum ascorbic acid, carotene, percent TPP effect . . . , and urinary thiamine and riboflavin.[30] The authors of the 1965 study conclude conservatively: "In particular, the daily intake of ascorbic acid, thiamine, and riboflavin needs to be increased; this means more fruits and vegetables from the harvest should be consumed, more milk and cheese incorporated into meals, and the possible use of enriched rice investigated. Some provision for making more than one meal a day available to field workers is necessary."[31]

Finally, in 1970 fifteen physicians spent four days in the lower Rio Grande Valley in Hidalgo County, Texas, under the auspices of the Field Foundation.[32] The purpose of their visit was, they readily admit, to discover a state of health among the poor farm workers in that area that would permit national attention to be drawn to them. Although the physicians had intended to conduct a survey of families, they were in fact invaded by over 900 persons wanting treatment. This the physicians provided, noting down their diagnoses. Although their bias is obvious and the procedure not a survey at all, each patient did have a rather thorough workup, and the results were impressive in the extent of the treatable pathology uncovered. They found the following conditions to be common: malnutrition; chronic skin disease; visual and hearing loss; intestinal parasitism; diabetes mellitus; thyroid disease; "multiple pregnancies syndrome"; very poor oral hygiene; uncorrected congenital deformities; no evidence of rehabilitation of persons with nerve injuries, fractures, or strokes; untreated seizures; multiple back deformities; active pulmonary tuberculosis; degenerative diseases of the heart and great vessels; and hypertension. Interestingly, anemia was uncommon. Not only was the level of health low, but so too was the level and amount of medical treatment.

In addition to physical ills, psychiatrist Robert Coles points out that the very fact of migrancy produces psychologic adaptations that, while "normal" under the circumstances, are joyless and in many ways pathetic. Lacking permanent residence, migrants even lack the neighborhood culture and institutions that other poor have. "There is a tendency to feel not only weak and hard pressed but responsible for that fate. Particularly unfortunate is such self-accusation when, in point of fact, these migrant families are willing to move about so far and wide, working so hard. . . . They are rootless, and for that reason sadder and more desperate than the sharecroppers I've studied or the mountain people of Appalachia."[33]

Migrants, in sum, seem to be much more ill, both chronically and acutely, than the large majority of Americans. Their specific pattern of diseases is not known, but they are probably subject to the same range of chronic illnesses as the majority of Americans, and, in addition, have superimposed on them the range of illnesses, both chronic and acute, that afflicted most Americans some years ago (e.g., infectious diseases), plus occupational diseases. Unscientifically, many observers think the hard work and deprivation that are the migrants' lot from early childhood make them old more quickly.

Despite their poor state of health, one would expect that the migrants would feel themselves more pressed to find proper food, clothing, and shelter than medical care. Nonetheless, in an East Coast survey, medical care was named most frequently as the service needed and received.[34] Unsurprisingly, it is women and children among migrants who consume the majority of health care.[35]

C. Federal Laws and Programs [36]

Federal legislation has rather often taken direct cognizance of the existence of migrant workers. In the 1930s, farm workers were explicitly exempted from the important labor laws passed, in deference to the lobbying power of the farm blocs; in the 1960s, explicit mention of farm workers in legislation was more frequently to their benefit, but their exclusion in the 1930s has not been fully rectified.

The agricultural workers' historical exclusion from (or only partial inclusion in) the nation's basic labor legislation is reflected in the National Labor Relations Act, which specifically exempted farm workers from its provisions.

> Some years ago, exclusion of farm workers from the Federal collective bargaining umbrella probably was mainly due to opposition from the farm bloc. Today the chief obstacle seems to be inability of supporters to agree upon and unite behind a single measure to bring coverage to agricultural labor.[37]

This inability stems from the fact that the farm workers have been able to make some progress in organizing without NLRA protection, and inclusion would entail restricting such current practices as secondary boycotting. Nonetheless, exclusion from the Act, since its original passage in 1935, discouraged labor union organization, and must certainly be counted as a severe disadvantage.

Agricultural labor is specifically exempted from coverage under the Federal Unemployment Tax Act of 1935.

The Fair Labor Standards Act (the Federal Wage and Hour Law), passed in 1938, excluded migrants completely until 1966, and now enforces no time-and-a-half overtime provision, and only a reduced minimum wage, and applies only to those farms large enough to employ seven full-time employees in any one quarter. This last provision will be of diminishing importance, since 3 percent of all farms now employ 60 percent of all hired labor on the farm, and the trend to large farm size continues.

The child labor provisions of the Fair Labor Standards Act are weaker than for non-agricultural industry; children of any age (as against at least fourteen years old off the farm) may work at non-hazardous jobs during non-school hours, and must be only sixteen years old (as against eighteen years old off the farm) for hazardous jobs. In fact, even these laws are regularly and shockingly violated.[37a]

Farm workers were included under Social Security only after 1951, and minimum criteria of receiving at least $150 from one employer or working for one employer at least twenty full days apply to agriculture, whereas no minimum limits at all apply off the farm.

The United States Employment Service, created in 1918 and continued by the Wagner-Peyser Act of 1933, operates the Department of Labor's Farm Labor Service through state employment offices, and is supposed to act as a benign matching service between farm and farm worker. In fact, investigators have found that the interests of the growers are consistently served, and the interests of the workers consistently undermined.[38] Growers utilizing the service are required to meet strong housing standards for their workers; enforcement of this statute is lax, however.

Even if the permanent laws passed in the 1930s neglected migrants, the terrible problems of rural dislocation during the depression did evoke a number of federal and state temporary expedient programs of relief, housing, and health. In an excellent but unpublished work,[39] Raymond C. Lerner has chronicled and analyzed how the acute crisis among displaced Okies and Arkies in California provoked only shabby treatment from the State Relief Organization, and passivity from the local and state health departments. The Farm Security Agency moved strongly to provide medical services for families in the federal camps and then elsewhere, establishing under California law in 1938 the Agricultural Workers Health and Medical Association. AWHMA lasted until 1947, when Congress voted to withdraw its support.

AWHMA was made politically viable by the fact that, as Lerner quotes a California Medical Association spokesman, "the migrant, due to lack of medical care, 'became a health menace to the citizens of California as well as a danger to himself. . . .'" The physicians were kept in charge of the program "with the right to choose a physician remaining inviolate."[40] The Board of Directors included four FSA officials, three physicians from the California Medical Association, the State Department of Public Health, and the State Relief Administration.

AWHMA service reached their peak in 1940–41 with a budget of $1.4 million and about 55,000 persons enrolled. It operated through acute diagnostic and treatment centers and referral centers, utilizing public health nurses at local AWHMA offices, and local physicians in their own offices.

> In 1940 FSA was still largely defending its action in entering the field of medical relief; by 1942 it was boldly proclaiming the fundamental contribution it had made, and should continue to make to the health and well-being of migratory farm labor. Initially, the AWHMA was conceived of as an organization designed to buy services for the destitute, utilizing the contract principle with local physicians, dentists, drug stores and hospitals; ultimately, before the whole structure was abandoned (by 1947) it had entered largely into the business of directly providing services through its own employed physicians and dispensaries.[41]

During the war the Okie problem in California ostensibly disappeared, migrant labor became Mexican and Mexican-American, and AWHMA was transferred to the War Food Administration and after the war to the Production and Marketing Administration of USDA. There being no acute crises in 1947, the program was killed. It was fifteen years later that the Migrant Health Program was born, as is related in the next chapter. Lerner states, "A glance at the types of programs to be established by these grants indicates that the experience with AWHMA has left its imprint."[42]

Not surprisingly, Lerner concludes:

> the views and actions taken (by the various agencies were) seldom based primarily on the medical or health needs of the migrants. . . . FSA people were concerned to maintain the viability of agriculture; California health officials wished to protect the resident population; welfare officials wished to restrict the relief rolls; organized medicine desired to protect itself from state medicine; the individual physician was obliged to earn a living and wished to limit the demand upon himself for medical charity; the liberals, intellectuals and humanitarians were concerned with reforming society in *order to save it*; New Dealers sought political victory; organized labor was not directly concerned. . . . the particular position taken on these issues by each party was clearly a function of the benefits resulting to each party. Thus, aid to the migrant was determined primarily by whether it benefitted the other fellow in a position to act, and secondly, if at all, by whether it benefited the migrant."[43]

In the 1930s laws, where the migrants would have needed no special mention to benefit, they got mentioned for the purpose of exclusion; in the 1960s laws, where the migrants would have needed special mention to benefit, they got no mention and so were often excluded. Nutrition legislation provides one example:

> . . . existing solutions to America's hunger problems, designed and administered for a stable population, are largely inapplicable and ineffective for migrants. Because they are constantly on the move, migrants do not have the non-governmental resources such as local credit or private charity normally provided by community to its residents. Yet none of the Federal, State, or local public assistance programs are designed to accommodate nonresident instream migrants.[44]

Medicaid provides another example. Title XIX of the Social Security Act passed in 1965, Medicaid is a federal and state medical assistance program for persons falling into certain defined categories, run by the individual states. Most migrants have not been covered by Medicaid for reasons they share with nonmigrants who are not eligible—chiefly, that although they are poor, they do not fall into one of the declared categories of persons who are aged, blind, or disabled, or in families with either an incapacitated or unemployed parent. Federal matching is not available under Medicaid for families headed by males working full time.

Beyond the categorical impediments, however, lie barriers particularly stringent for migrants. Most importantly, to be covered by a state's Medicaid program, a person must be able to declare that he intends to be a permanent resident of the state in question. Only in emergencies, moreover, can an out-of-state facility receive reimbursement from the home state Medicaid agency. The very fact of migrancy, then, is a hindrance if the categorical criteria are met in the first place.

A second hindrance is the manner in which income is determined. (After it has been determined that a family meets the category test, it must be established that the family's income is below a certain state-determined level.) Documentation of income must be produced, which in itself is difficult for migrants who work for many different employers and for whom paper work is often not done.

The usual method of income determination calls for establishment of recent income and extrapolation of that for a yearly level. Migrants, however, are without work for long periods of time, and extrapolation is not valid for them.

Other hindrances to migrant eligibility for Medicaid are the language barrier, which impedes the process of eligibility determination and registration, and the unfortunate fact that the home states of many migrants are Florida and Texas, which have only minimal Medicaid coverage, and Arizona, which until recently has had no program at all.

Several of the federal agencies—the Community Health Service, the Medical Services Administration, which administers Medicaid, and others—have recognized the problems involved here and have proposed various solutions, but as yet none have been implemented.

The Control Systems Research, Inc., survey of migrants in Homestead found a surprisingly large percentage categorically eligible for Medicaid (residency, income, and other state requirements not considered): 48 percent of the 66 black families, and 19 percent of the 420 Chicano families. Of these, however, only three black and five Chicano families were actually receiving Medicaid.[45]

In recent years, some programs have at last had special provisions added to enable migrants to partake of the benefits. Of four standards set by the Occupational Safety and Health Act of 1970, one regulating construction and sanitation standards for temporary labor camps is applicable to migrants. Unfortunately, whereas all industry-wide standards under OSHA are applicable to all industries where they in fact apply, agriculture forms an exception. So machinery guarding and shielding standards apply wherever that machinery is used except on a farm, ladder regulations apply in all areas except farms, and movable toilets are provided where work requires it except on a farm.

Still, OSHA's housing standards are generally similar to those of the Wagner-Peyser Act and stronger than most of the states' statutes. If enforced, probably no further standards would be necessary to ensure the migrants decent housing. That enforcement requires first a complaint from an afflicted person, to be followed by OSHA administration inspection, seems at present the major block to widespread housing improvement. Were an organization active in informing the workers of their rights and forwarding complaints to OSHA, conformity with the law might be swifter, but such is not the case.

Non-agricultural industry has had occupational safety standards for many years, so OSHA was able to take them over fairly readily. Since the farm has been essentially unregulated, there has been an understandable delay in formulating standards; the strength of the farm lobby has also added delay. Some progress has been made, however, in two fields, and there is hope for progress in a third.

In 1972 OSHA was petitioned by the Migrant Legal Action Program to promulgate pesticide standards, which they did on an emergency basis. After much lobbying and legal maneuvering by the farm bloc and MLAP, a good standard was permanently adopted. The Environmental Protection Agency also promulgated standards for pesticide exposure, but they are fairly weak.

Farm safety equipment is also coming to be regulated. Although permanent standards are not yet adopted, tractor roll-over, machinery guarding, and personal protective equipment, noise, and nuisance dust regulations are all being considered. Although OSHA has rejected setting immediate standards for field sanitation—toilets, drinking water, and washing facilities—on the grounds that other work takes priority, they will probably take this issue up soon.

OSHA, then, offers some real assistance to migrants in an important area. The main problem in the near future will probably be enforcement of such standards as are promulgated, since a local presence to identify deficiencies is needed but lacking.

The operations of farm labor contractors are weakly regulated by the Farm Labor Contractor Registration Act, although some rights of laborers are thereby protected.[46] The Interstate Commerce Act has authorized the Federal Highway Administration to set standards for the interstate transportation of migrant workers.

Title V of the Housing Act of 1949 was amended in 1961 to enable the Farmers Home Administration of the USDA "to provide safe, decent, and sanitary housing facilities for domestic farm laborers through insured loan programs and low-rent housing grant programs." In 1973 the loan appropriation was $10.2 million, the grant appropriation was $1.7 million.

The Department of Labor's Manpower Development and Training Act has had special money set aside for the purpose of helping migrant workers convert from seasonal to full-time employment. The Emergency Employment Act of 1971 enables states to apply for federal aid for transitional employment in public service jobs and for job training program funds. Migrant farm workers and seven other categories of workers are to receive priority for funds. Title III-B of the Economic Opportunity Act, passed in 1965, has funded local projects for migrants in four fields of endeavor: reemployment and adjustment assistance, education and training, permanent housing, and in-stream assistance (1974 appropriation—$40 million). In 1967 an amendment to Title I of the Elementary and Secondary Education Act enabled direct or supplementary education projects for migrants to be funded (1974 appropriation $78 million).

Only with the social legislation binge of the 1960s did the migrants get positive recognition from the federal government. But the basic problem of exemption from the fundamental legislation of the 1930s remained.

D. State Laws

The states have passed laws in such areas as minimum wage, collection of wages, working hours, child labor, working conditions, labor contractors, collective bargaining, workmen's compensation, unemployment compensation, housing, health, and education. Provisions vary from state to state, but no state in fact offers a great deal of significant aid to the farm worker. Table 1-3 shows how little has been done at the state level, and even then the case is overstated in the states' favor, since many of the laws frequently go unenforced.

Of most direct significance to health are the laws on housing. The state and local health departments are generally entrusted with the responsibility of inspecting camps and other worker housing for sanitary facilities, showers, water, sometimes screening, and the like. Although usually weaker than Wagner-Peyser or OSHA requirements, the laws would likely have a significant effect in improving health if they were enforced.

As with federal medical programs, state and county medical care for indigents often manages to miss the migrant. Greenfield found in a 1961 mail survey in California that

> Residence requirements are a definite hindrance in giving hospital care to migratory farm workers except in a medical emergency. Of the 35 counties that are heavy employers of such labor, only 15 will give service to someone who has State but not county residence, and only 9 of these will serve an individual who has neither state nor county residence. For the most part, service is given only during the period of investigation and authorization to return to legal residence, or when the applicant has expressed an intent to reside in the county.[47]

Anecdotal reports universally support the impression that the California situation is typical of other states as well.

E. Summary

Migrant workers, then, number approximately 172,000 themselves, or as many as one million including families, are most young, mostly black or Chicano, have low educational achievements, bad housing and environment, and

Table 1-3. State Laws

	Calif.	*Colo.*	*Fla.*	*Ill.*	*Mich.*	*N.J.*	*N.Y.*	*Ore.*	*Tex.*	*Wash.*
Workmen's Compensation	OK	No	partial	partial	partial	elective	OK	OK	No	OK
Minimum Wage	OK	No	No	OK	OK	OK	OK	fair	fair	No
Work Hours	No	No	10/day	No	No	No	No	No	No	No
Child Labor	fair	fair	poor	No	No	OK	OK	fair	poor	poor
Working Conditions	minimal	No	No	No	No	minimal	No	No	minimal	No
Collective Bargaining	fair-poor	No	No	No	No	OK	OK	fair	No	fair
Unemployment Compensation	temp. disabil.	No	No	No	No	No	No	No	No	No

very low incomes. Their state of health is remarkably poor, but data are inadequate to delineate specifically incidences and prevalences of their diseases.

While the federal government excluded farm workers from the permanent labor laws of the 1930s, temporary depression programs were supplied. The Agricultural Workers Health and Medical Association was a precursor of the 1962 Migrant Health Act, following which the migrants were included in many Great Society programs. The provisions of the Occupational Safety and Health Act of 1970 will have important benefits for migrants. Many laws still find migrants excluded de facto if not de jure, however, and they have not been included in the basic laws of the 1930s as yet. The state laws offer little solace.

II PROBLEMS OF RURAL HEALTH CARE

A. General Description

In rural areas, as elsewhere in America, the health care system is divided into two spheres, private and public. Generally, the private system has had its pick of what services to offer. Those items foregone by the private system have fallen into the realm of public agencies.

Local health departments carry the burden of environmental sanitation, certain preventive medicine measures, and certain kinds of nursing services to the poor in rural areas. County hospitals also provide some medical services for the indigent.

The county has handled environmental sanitation, waste disposal, water supply, restaurant sanitation, etc., pretty well for the non-poor community. But, just as metropolitan governments have served non-slum areas preferentially, in rural areas water supplies to poor areas are polluted, housing codes go unenforced, and environmental sanitation is generally neglected.

Preventive medical services offered by county health departments serve primarily the poor. They fall into two categories: clinics for certain infectious diseases that would constitute a threat to the entire community if the poor were allowed to harbor them—tuberculosis, venereal disease, and the immunizable diseases—and clinics for mothers and children—well-baby, family planning, maternal and infant health, prenatal, etc.

Health departments usually provide public health nursing and health education services, too. The nurses staff the categorical clinics, visit homes of poor families with medical care problems, and often try to fend within the existing system for families that come to their attention. Health education can consist of community-wide campaigns on several issues and/or personal education services delivered in homes or at the clinic.

Despite these activities, health departments are not the major institutions responsible for preventive medicine in a community. For one thing, they deal almost exclusively with those who cannot afford private practitioners, who also give immunizations, prescribe birth control pills, etc. For another, health departments deal almost exclusively in primary prevention (preventing a disease from occurring), whereas private medicine deals with both primary and secondary prevention. The latter consists of early disease detection and preventive supervision; examples would be periodic physical examinations, advice on weight reduction, and control of high blood pressure.

Finally, the public sector provides medical care for the poor in county hospitals. The deficiencies of city and county hospitals are by now well known. Rural hospitals are just as inadequate as urban hospitals in this respect, even worse in that few outpatient services are offered, even inadequate ones.

The private sector of medical care is of course the more prestigious in the United States. Until recently, it was often claimed (particularly by organized medicine) that there was a "mainstream of medical care" dispensed primarily by the private system, and that care was available to all, rich or poor, alike. Significantly, these claims are now heard less often, even from organized medicine. Most now acknowledge the inability of the system to deliver care even to all who can pay, let alone those who cannot. This supply problem derives from, first, a manpower shortage, and second, an organization of care that seems rather inefficient.

The simple facts of manpower are that there are many more physicians per capita in urban America than in rural America. Although 30 percent of the people in America reside in the rural areas, those areas have only 12 percent of the physicians, 18 percent of the nurses, 14 percent of the pharmacists, 8 percent of the pediatricians, and 4 percent of the psychiatrists.[48] In addition, the rural areas have predominantly general practitioners with an older average age than all doctors. Quality of care is thought to be adversely affected by these factors. The clear implication, then, is that there are too few physicians in rural areas to do the same kind of job as is done in urban areas.

The organization of medical care in rural areas seems to be but little different from that in urban areas. Although physicians are organized in groups in rural areas more than elsewhere, the predominant form is still individual solo practice, and this can be particularly difficult for the rural physician:

> In the larger cities, physicians have increasingly come to share office facilities and the urban "medical arts building" has promoted communications between doctors even when they are in separate quarters. The busy urban hospital is a further channel for interchange. The relative isolation of the rural or small town doctor, by contrast, deprives him of the stimulation necessary to keep abreast of the endless advances in medical science.[49]

The complaints about this system of care can be looked at in two ways. First, the services that physicians traditionally deliver are quite possibly delivered more efficiently by groups than by individuals, especially when financial arrangements specify prepayment rather than fee-for-service. General economic theory, as explained by Fein,[50] indicates that groups should benefit by economies of scale not attainable by solo practitioners—physicians and intermediate level health personnel are more able to specialize in groups, and often indivisible economic units can be used more fully. Theory also "indicates that *prepaid* practice is expected to be more efficient than fee-for-service practice, in terms of avoidance of unnecessary utilization of expensive procedures. Research, to date, has not effectively proven these reasonable hypotheses to be false."[51] On the other hand, research has not proven them to be true. Second, solo practice delivers only traditional services, whereas group practices with vertical integration of services can supply such services as home nursing care, transportation, and preventive screening examinations that would be quite difficult to arrange otherwise. In a sense this second criticism is on the grounds of efficiency, too. Medical care is really a series of services that are to some extent dependent on one another. Prevention, diagnosis, outpatient treatment, inpatient treatment, and rehabilitation are interlinked for many diseases. Removing any links in the chain leads to services that must be provided somewhere else along the chain, or to ill health. For instance, if the only services offered were diagnosis and inpatient treatment, many inefficient situations would obviously result. Roemer and Anzel state that this very situation is probably quite common in rural areas, leading to high hospitalization rates per outpatient visit.[52] Since the solo physician is less frequently in a position to provide all the services along the chain, or to arrange for them, than a well-organized multispecialty group practice, solo practice leads to systematic inefficiency.

In fact, group practice is not the only answer for the second complaint about solo practice. Another system that might serve just as well would be found by a series of interlinked companies. The same principle makes it possible for the software and hardware services of a computer company to be divorced. Actually, then, the second criticism of solo practice condemns not solo practice, but the overall system arrangements in rural areas.

Medical care facilities are not such a problem. Thanks largely to the Hill-Burton program begun just after World War II, the number of hospital beds in rural areas is comparable to those in urban areas on a per capita basis. The quality of the medicine practiced in them has been questioned however; a major emphasis of the Regional Medical Programs legislation was to disperse knowledge and practice currently available in the metropolitan centers out to the periphery. Hospitals in rural areas tend to be smaller than in urban areas, and the quality of smaller hospitals is no doubt below that of larger ones. There is a relative shortage of nursing home beds in rural areas. But, in general, facilities are not a major stumbling block in rural health care.

Both the rural middle class and the rural poor have been affected by the medical care services shortage; increasing demand and decreasing supply in recent years have multiplied complaints from both sectors. Most complaints from the middle class cite increased appointment delays, decreased quality of services (decreased time per visit), and increased price. The usual remedy suggested by the complainants is increasing the supply of physicians; the poor add complaints of discrimination on both ethnic and economic bases.

B. Changes in Rural Health Services

Even in the face of manifest and increasing dissatisfaction, there have been few changes in rural medical manpower and organization. Manpower production has not been automatically responsive to increased needs in the rural areas and elsewhere because the production units (medical schools, in the case of physicians) are not tied directly to service production. That is, if the institution can produce more physicians (and other manpower) who can subsequently become productive, it results in no significant financial profit for that institution, nor have any other incentives influenced them to increase their production.

Manpower distribution has had a certain responsiveness to current trends that manpower production has not, but this has hurt the rural areas. More mobile than most of the population, the physicians have been free to follow the general trend of population into the cities and suburbs, predominantly the latter. Beyond the usual attractions of the city, special medical sector influences have concentrated physicians there. The modern emphasis on specialization and consequent reliance on institutions and their special equipment have been important. The schools themselves, almost always located in metropolitan areas, have admitted students with predominantly urban backgrounds. Finally, the "doctor shortage" together with the relative wealth of the cities and suburbs have provided physicians with financial incentives to remain in metropolitan areas.

The system of medical care delivery has remained stagnant for several reasons. First of all, there have been few forces pushing hard for change. Third party payers have not pushed, and consumers have not pushed until recently—and they are more interested in simply getting more physicians than changing the system. Secondly, although it would seem likely that medical care providers would be able to reap more financial profit with less effort through reorganization, this likelihood is not proved. Moreover, loss of non-corporate and independent existence is a potent disincentive to physicians. The general conservativeness of the profession is enhanced by the fact that most rural practitioners are older, and their personal cost of change of habit therefore increased. They already make good money, so the financial improvement foreseen would have to be clear and marked for change to come. In addition, long work hours have come to have a certain positive valuation in the profession, so saving some of them is an ambiguous benefit. Finally, the use of intermediate level health personnel has been retarded by state laws, malpractice insurance requirements, and by the scarcity of such persons. Given this system of incentives, it is not hard to understand why new modes of organization of medical practice in rural areas have not flourished.

Since spontaneous adjustment in the marketplace did not work, the federal government and others have tried to solve the rural medical care problem directly. Five separate types of attempts can be discerned.

One of the oldest solutions was offered by the Hill-Burton Program of hospital building. It is not clear whether lack of hospital facilities was ever a bottleneck for good quality and quantity medical care in rural areas or not. At present, certainly, the hospital problem is not the major one. Direct federal subsidy of hospital construction through this program has seen to that.

The most obvious point of attack has been the attraction of physicians to rural areas. One approach has been the establishment of new medical schools in the rural states, such as Kentucky, West Virginia, and New Mexico. The results of this approach have been disappointing; even though favorite sons are favored for admission, various factors have conspired to make almost negligible the effects these schools have had on increasing rural physician manpower.

Another approach to manpower attraction has been constructing modern office facilities and recruiting physicians to come use them with inviting financial terms. Small towns, either on their own or from 1959 until recently with the help of the Sears-Roebuck Foundation, have tried this approach, and the AMA has helped them by trying to locate the physicians. One service the Foundation offered was performance of a community survey to assess the economic feasibility of supporting a physician in the area in question. Service to the poor was not a prime aim of the Foundation. The Foundation stopped its activities in this field recently, however, when a survey showed that a great many of the communities it helped had subsequently lost the doctor and lapsed back into their previous situation.

Another approach tried by some southern states has been to subsidize a medical student's education, and forgive the loan in repayment for rural service. "Virginia's State Health Commissioner, however, comments: 'It is hard to evaluate the effectiveness of the program. Certainly it has not been a great boon to (medical) practice in the rural areas; on the other hand, it has helped fill a monetary need for these students'."[53]

Recently, the Student American Medical Association sponsored a summer in Appalachia for some medical students, hoping to attract them to the area permanently. Although all enjoyed the summer working with the practitioners in the area, less than 10 percent thought they might consider returning there for any length of time.

A third approach is for the federal government to employ directly the necessary personnel, and simply assign them to an area. The Indian Health

Service has supplied health care services to the American Indians directly for many years, using facilities and personnel that are wholly federal.

A variant on this approach is taken by the National Health Service Corps, created by the Emergency Health Personnel Act of 1970. Under its provisions, health personnel may be employed by the Public Health Service and assigned to areas with critical health manpower shortages. As of January 1, 1974, 336 persons are so assigned. Madison described the strategy of the National Health Service Corps as follows:

> The term 'emergency' was used to signify the belief that the problem is a temporary one, or that the National Health Service Corps is an 'emergency' rather than a permanent solution. Whether or not this belief is justified, the Corps relies on two new strategies that have not been widely used before in this country: (1) *indirect conscription*—an organized corps that can assign health professionals to communities within a framework of support—both financial and professional—thus alleviating some of the risks inherent in the usual entrepreneurship approach used by physicians and dentists when locating in small communities; and (2) *community process for structuring a setting* within which primary health care can be delivered. Whether these two strategies will work remains to be seen; however, both are elements that have generally been lacking in the past. The importance of adequate professional support to the choice of a young physician to practice in a rural area (or anywhere else) is now taken as a given, while the significance of achieving wide community involvement and commitment in attempting to solve a community's health care problems has also been widely called for and is now judged by many to be crucially important to a successful effort.[54]

The NHSC has not been in existence long enough to gauge its success as a model. By its goals and scope, however, one can predetermine that in and of itself it can have but little impact on the health personnel maldistribution problem.

A fourth approach to rural health problems has been through attempts at rationalization. The basic idea behind regionalization is to distribute the quality and in some cases quantity of medical care available in urban centers to more isolated areas. Some voluntary agreements between small, rural hospitals and larger, more urban ones have been consummated in the past, but little of substance has come of them.[55] The Hill-Burton legislation had elements of regional planning in it, and it was successful in assuring that highly specialized operations would be confined to urban areas, and that more rural than urban beds would be supplied. The Regional Medical Programs have concentrated, since their inception in 1965, on supplying education and consultation to outlying centers. Beyond that, little has really been obtained. None of these programs has been successful enough to either attract manpower or to change the system of care in rural areas; indeed, it is questionable if there has been any change in the quality of that care that is delivered.

Fifth, there have been some attempts at organizational change in rural areas. The United Mine Workers in Appalachia created a system of hospitals and group practices that served their constituents well and efficiently, and even served to attract personnel to the area. The uniqueness of that situation obviously lay in the strong union built by John L. Lewis. Today, the system has decayed, and most of the hospitals have been sold to independent groups.

The neighborhood health center movement, another attempt at reorganization, has not left the rural scene untouched. Although the Office of Economic Opportunity spent most of its money on urban areas, the Office of Health Affairs did initiate several rural health centers, in the Southeast and Appalachia for its most successful efforts. Whether or not neighborhood health centers in general, or the rural ones in specific, improve the productivity of the doctor is unclear. It is said that NHC's are geared to deliver so many types of services in an integrated package it has been impossible to allocate costs for the specific services a general practitioner or even a group practice would deliver, especially in light of the newness of NHC's and their expected large startup costs. Many further unanswered questions remain.

Madison has speculated that the issues of manpower recruitment and organizational change are intimately intertwined. He has tried to show, in an as yet unpublished study, that rural communities retain physicians in proportion to the extent to which medical practice in the community is explicitly organized. Such recently started efforts as Health Maintenance Organizations and the manpower programs mentioned in Chapter 5, Part III, would thus be seen to have important rural consequences, if Madison is correct.

It should also be mentioned, finally, that passage of health insurance bills by the federal government might well have important effects on rural medical care, depending on the specific provisions. Voluntary health insurance and Medicare and Medicaid in the past have had no such discernible effect, however, that has been demonstrated.

C. Summary

Rural area public sector health services consist of environmental sanitation, categorical clinics, public health nursing, health education, and hospital services delivered by the county health departments and hospitals. The poor are often ill-served by this sector. The private sector of personal health care is acknowledged to be unable to handle the heavy demands placed on it, and suffers from manpower deficiency and possibly organizational inefficiency problems. Facilities, although promoting generally low quality care, are not regarded as a major bottleneck. Automatic adjustment of manpower and organizational problems has not occurred through a market or other automatic mechanism.

Five different solutions to rural health problems have been tried: hospital building; attraction of physician manpower by new state medical schools, building of office facilities and invitation, student subsidy, and rural experience in medical school; direct federal service; regional associations; and direct building of a new system on limited bases. None has proved very successful as yet, but new federal manpower programs and efforts to promote Health Maintenance Organizations will have implications for the future—particularly if it is true that more tightly organized medical care systems tend to retain physicians fairly well in rural areas.

III THE PROBLEM OF MIGRANT HEALTH—CAUSATION

The background data presented in this chapter can be combined with a general knowledge of disease causation to construct a chain of causality for the poor state of the health of migrants (see fig. 1-4). Unfortunately, although figure 1-4 seems eminently reasonable, medical knowledge is not sufficiently advanced, and the epidemiology of the diseases of migrants not sufficiently well delineated, to enable us to establish with scientific rigor or to quantify any of the relationships. We cannot quantify the connection between a specific cause and result—e.g., to what extent (and with what coexistent conditions) crowded housing leads to respiratory infections—nor can we quantify how much of what kind of diseases would be relieved by a single correction made—e.g., how much relief of which diseases we would be buying by ensuring a decrease of crowding in the camps.

Rough as it is, however, it would seem more foolish to reject this reasonable scheme of causality than to accept it, and it is useful, too, in classifying various approaches to the problem and in providing rough estimates of their probable effectiveness.

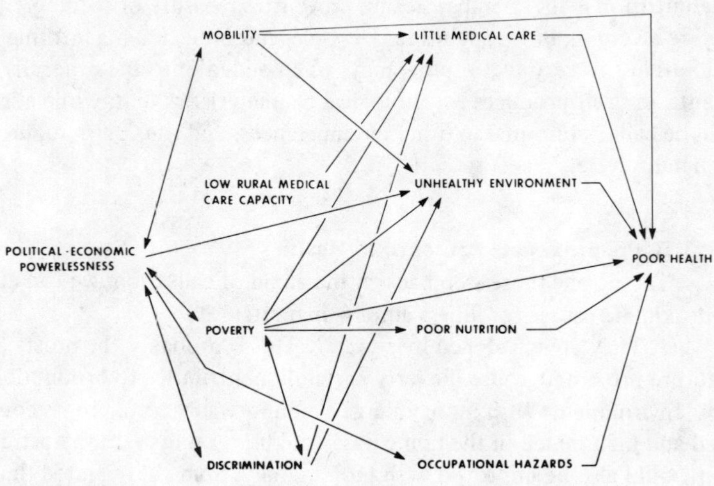

Figure 1-4. Causal Scheme of Poor Health among Migrants.

A. Proximate Causes of Ill Health

Five proximate causes for illness among migrants can be cited:

1. They obtain *little medical care.* Being human, the migrants suffer from genetic diseases (diabetes), happenstance diseases (cancer), degenerative diseases (heart disease), and other diseases to which all flesh is heir–urinary tract infections, congential defects, etc. These diseases are subject to the ministrations of medical care, including early detection, preventive supervision, treatment, and rehabilitation. Yet, the Homestead survey found that 50 percent of families made no physician visits in a year, and 70 percent spent less than $100 on medical expenses. The pattern of seeking medical care was illness or injury oriented, generally at a hospital emergency room, hospital outpatient clinic, or private doctor's office.[56]
2. They are subjected to *detrimental environmental influences.* Poor and crowded housing, bad water, poor sanitation around the homes and in the fields lead to increased incidence of acute infectious diseases, and chronic ones such as tuberculosis. Such diseases are most amenable to primary prevention–removal of the agent alleviates the disease incidence–but can also be subject to medical treatment.
3. They are subjected to *detrimental occupational influences.* The accident rate of farm labor is high, exposure to pesticides is a chronic and acute problem, and the severe nature of the work leads to overexhaustion, general susceptibility to disease, arthritis, and most likely "premature ageing." Here again, primary prevention is the approach of choice, but medical care provision is also applicable.
4. They are a *malnourished* population. Although malnutrition is a disease in itself, it also leads a susceptibility to other diseases. The preferred approach to malnutrition is the therapeutic and preventive measure of feeding.
5. They are a very *mobile* population. Dr. Coles has indicated his informed opinion that this very fact of migrancy, when added onto the other ills of the migrants, in itself produces psychological characteristics that, while adaptive, would be called abnormal in other circumstances, and thus perpetuates the migrant cycle.

B. Pre-proximate Causes of Ill Health

Taking one more step back in the chain of causation; we can cite five pre-proximate causes for illness among migrants:

1. They are enveloped by *poverty*. This is probably the most important pre-proximate cause. Poverty certainly contributes to production of an unhealthy environment. With money, larger and more substantial units could be purchased and maintained in the home base, and better units rented upstream. Nutrition would also be improved with more money. Some have stated that

nutritional education is the necessary ingredient, but more studies have shown that indigent consumers most often make "good" choices of food when they have sufficient money to spend. Specifically for migrants, in the Colorado Migrant Council study of nutrition, it was found that "When the additional money was available for food, the mothers reported they purchased more meat, milk, fruit (apples, bananas, oranges), and vegetables (tomatoes, lettuce) in that order. If less money was available, these foods would be cut out in the reverse order. . . . Money is not available for adequate health care or nutrition." [57] A further effect of poverty is the inability to purchase medical care.

2. *Rural medical care delivery capacity* is insufficient. That this assertion is true in general has been indicated in the previous section; the Community Change, Inc., study very nicely showed how it is specifically true for the migrant impact counties [58] (see table 1-4). Taking 1 to 1,635 as the national average ratio of primary care physicians to population, and 1 to 2,509 as the average rural ratio, they called any county's ratio adequate if it were better than 1 to 1,635, substandard if it fell between 1 to 1,636 and 1 to 2,509, and critical if it were worse than that. Table 1-4 shows that both home-base and upstream counties have about as many better than the rural average as worse. The more favorable picture from the mixed counties perhaps reflects the predominance in that category of counties in well-doctored California. Most migrant areas are clearly deficient in manpower.

If medical care were more readily available in rural areas, the migrant would still have trouble getting it, given the other factors we are here considering. Nonetheless, if medical care were more readily available—and were of good enough quality that it were worthwhile to purchase it—when the migrant could surmount the other obstacles, he would be more able to get it. In addition, were rural medical care more available, the prices might be more acceptable.

3. *The mobility of the migrant.* Mobility leads to ineligibility for the various usually meager social welfare programs that exist, and thus perpetuates poverty to some extent. It leads to an inability to ferret out medical care in the

Table 1-4. Primary Physicians in Migrant Impact Counties

Ratio of Primary Physicians to Population	*Type of County*			
	Home Base	*Mixed*	*Upstream*	*Total*
Adequate*	0	5	1	6
Substandard**	11	13	7	31
Critical***	10	3	9	22
Total	21	21	17	59

*1-1,635, better than the national average
**1,636-2,509, better than the rural average
***2,510-, worse than the rural average
Source: Community Change, Inc.

unfamiliar (and insufficient) channels upstream. Mobility also leads to a decreased influence of the migrants on the health departments and other governmental bodies upstream, not that the other poor upstream or they themselves downstream have much influence with the government. Mobility also decreases the chance for self-help environmental effects. The benefits gained would be short-lived.

4. *Discrimination against the migrant.* The poor are discriminated against in our society, as are minority groups, and most probably migrants *qua* migrants, although it is hard to tell, since all migrants are also poor. This discrimination in all likelihood detracts from the quality and quantity of medical care available to migrants. Anecdotes abound on the subject of indignities heaped upon migrants not only by physicians, but by all types of Anglo or white personnel, such as nurses and receptionists. Hospitals are also noted for their suspicious ways with migrants, although a great deal of this behavior is no doubt associated with the financial barriers.

Discrimination is probably another factor contributing to the unhealthy environment the migrants live in. Once again, one can only intuit what the actual contribution of prejudice is to the horrible camps and lax enforcement, when there are also economic and political factors one could cite as causal. But that prejudice exists is abundantly clear to anyone who has talked to the parties in question; one must conclude that prejudice must have some effect on actions, and must not be merely a rationalizing ideology for deeds already done.

Finally, the interconnection with poverty is also a significant factor. As with health and poverty, the poor get discriminated against, and the objects of discrimination get poor. Operationally, this means that a well paying permanent job tends to get assigned to the non-migrant, and among the migrants, to whites and Anglos. Once again, although this point is not formally documented, every dispassionate observer in the field knows that the point is valid.

5. The *lack of political influence* of the migrant. Most specifically we refer here to county governments. As a result, though county governments contribute to irrigation pipelines, the same governments are unwilling to appropriate money for drinking water pipelines to the poor colonias in South Texas. Political powerlessness permits the existence of the low tax rates that prevent counties from substantial collections from the larger farms, which funds could be used in turn for environmental purposes such as those we have mentioned. Health department sanitarians are understandably unwilling to put legal muscle behind requests for corrections of violations, when the action would be taken against the same growers who directly or indirectly control the very Board of County Supervisors that employs the health officer and sanitarian.[59] Upstream this lack of political influence is related to mobility, but in the home-base areas it is related as well to poverty (impoverished groups all over seem unable to implement significant political changes), certain prejudicial practices, such as literacy tests, and the Texas legislated practice of purging the voter registration

lists annually, so that voter registration drives must be mounted each year *de novo*.

Lying behind these five pre-proximate cuases of ill health is the seminal cause of political-economic powerlessness at all levels, as documented by the Senate Subcommittee on Migratory Labor sixteen volume set of hearings on "Migrant and Seasonal Farmworkers Powerlessness." Although ultimate causes are hard to come by, many forces buttressing the status quo are identified there, and the fact that the migrants are indeed powerless emerges as indisputable. In our chart (fig. 1–4) we indicate a reciprocal relationship between political-economic powerlessness and mobility, poverty, and discrimination.

C. Red Herrings

Four explanations commonly offered for this migrants' poor state of health are really quite minor points. They are considered here for the purpose of perspective.

1. *Mobility leads to a lack of continuity of medical care.* Although continuity of medical care is of course lacking as migrants move from place to place, at present this is about a third order question. They get medical care at all only very infrequently, upstream or home base. Moreover, when medical care is obtained in home-base areas, continuity is frequently lacking even in that one stationary place—neither the type of continuity with a continuous record and different doctors, nor the type of continuity with the same doctor time after time with a proper record at hand. (This situation occurs because of the nature of the referral process, that taps many doctors for referrals, and the quality of the clinics, with few records.) It is true that public health nurses sometimes provide an admirable point of continuity of care, and sometimes, to be sure, physician continuity does exist, but most often the patient does not even get to see a doctor. Clearly, then, continuity along the stream is not a primal reason for ill health.

Furthermore, although continuity of care is certainly desirable, in many cases it does not make that much difference. With management of chronic diseases, continuity is often important. But with the common, acute diseases, not having seen the patient before is no barrier for the physician in rendering immediate and accurate treatment.

Difficulty in establishing continuity of care along a stream of migration will probably be a priority problem someday, but that day will be a welcome one, for at that point the task of delivering medical care services of acceptable quantity and quality for a large number of persons will have been accomplished.

2. *Public health personal preventive services are not extended to enough persons.* It is true that it might be helpful to have more persons served with well-baby clinics, VD and TB clinics, immunization clinics, and family planning clinics. We have noted previously, however, that the most important

functions served by the health departments lie in the field of environmental protection, and that the great bulk of personal health services are rendered by the private sector, both preventive and curative. The personal health services delivered by the public sector reflect the inability or unwillingness of the private sector to render them and the desire of the community at large to be protected from epidemics, not the virtue of these particular measures for the people treated. In other words, given a choice between the personal health services rendered by health departments and the personal health services rendered by the private sector, there is little reason to choose the former.

Moreover, public health departments deliver these services in categorical clinics, serving the convenience of the providers, but decidedly not that of consumers. The private sector services, where a family can be treated in one stop for all the ills afflicting it (within the limits of the capability of the particular provider), is a much more efficient operation overall, given that all services are to be rendered. It has never been shown that health department rendered services are particularly cost-efficient, and indeed it is unlikely that this is the case.

Well-baby clinics may serve as education devices, but they are fairly meaningless if there is little or no ability to take care of the patient once a defect has been uncovered. Although venereal disease is probably as prevalent among the migrant population as any other population, and treatment is certainly desirable, there are no particular efficiencies of scale to be obtained from having a special clinic just for that, and the diseconomies from a categorical clinic to the patient still apply. Furthermore, there is little to distinguish treatment of venereal disease from treatment of some other disease, such as a common urinary tract infection, as far as the individual patient is concerned. The question must naturally arise, therefore, why segregate care of this particular disease, if all the contact follow-ups could be as well handled in some other more comprehensive format?

Tuberculosis is more widespread among migrants than other groups, but once again there is no particular reason to provide care for this disease outside of a general treatment format. The great majority of cases can be handled by a competent internist; few need specialty consultation. No evidence leads us to suppose, moreover, that treatment of tuberculosis has a uniquely high payoff for the population in question, although it certainly should be treated.

The common immunizations offered, against polio, diphtheria, pertussis, tetanus, measles, mumps, and rubella, are of course desirable. Many of these diseases can cause mortality and severe morbidity. The whole process of immunizing would have to be very, very cheap to everyone concerned for emphasis on this phase to be very cost-effective, however, for these diseases, with the exception of measles, mumps and rubella, are decidedly rare, and the *total* mortality and morbidity not high. (Even though many persons rightly become indignant when the only cases of polio reported in 1969 occurred in South Texas among farm workers, there were very few persons involved.)

Family planning clinics alone seem to have some acceptable rationale for being offered. The services offered are very widely applicable, there is a good economy of scale to be obtained by periodically employing a specialist to prescribe medications and insert IUDs, and health education on this specific subject would be greatly enhanced by centralized application. Furthermore, there seems to be good reason to have group discussion sessions on this subject. But of course, all these reasons would be equally applicable in a comprehensive care setting.

In sum, although each of the services here examined would be desirable, it seems quite unlikely that these services would be the ones one would pick as being the most cost-effective, and one would certainly not choose that they be delivered in the categorical clinics that most health departments currently utilize.

3. *Migrants need more health education.* Of course everyone could use more health education. It is quite probable that the migrants' state of knowledge of disease causation is not high (although it is debatable how much different it is from that of the middle class), and that their knowledge of healthful sanitary practices is not great. This being agreed to, it is still far from clear that improving health education would be a useful step. We have already cited the Colorado Migrant Council study that indicates that lack of money, rather than ignorance, leads to malnutritious diets.[60] The sanitation problems are likewise fixed on an economic basis; the horrible conditions migrants live in did not appear because people did not know any better. Washing one's hands before eating does not make up for fecal drainage into the house. As for medical care, the important element here is access to professional health personnel; do-it-yourself medical care has not been proved a fruitful mode of delivery anywhere in the world. It would be useful for a mother to know the proper way to treat an infant with diarrhea; it would be safer and surer for her to have access to health professionals to make a diagnosis and prescribe treatment.

4. *Migrants need to be motivated to seek medical care.* The general question of motivation among migrants has been spoken to by Robert Coles. ". . . most of these people display an initiative and desire for work in striking contrast to their poor brethren in cities, ... Migrant farmworkers, almost by definition, show a remarkable capacity and desire to travel far and wide in search of work."[61] No migrant health project has ever reported a failure to fully utilize its services, although many stress the importance of outreach efforts. Even the new, large projects recently begun by the Migrant Health Program have had no problem recruiting patients. A study sponsored by the National Institutes of Health compared migrant camps with and without health clinics. "The results dramatically indicate that occupants in camps with clinics sought and received

medical attention significantly more frequently than occupants of camps without clinics."[62] The control figures of that study are especially interesting: in the camps without clinics 43 percent of the residents had received medical care for an injury or illness, and 40 percent had received complete immunizations. Motivation seems an unlikely bottleneck.

Moreover, it has been found time and time again in urban poor areas that the reasons for non-utilization of available resources have been: unavailable transportation, problems with child care, fragmented clinics, abrasive incidents with personnel, and finances. Usually in fact, poor people value medical care too much, and *over*-utilization of resources is a common problem, despite the disincentives.

D. Two Observations on the Causal Pattern

1. Many of the causes of poor health among migrants would seem to be true for the rural poor as well; only the problem of mobility is really unique to the migrants. Although the migrants are probably the worst off among the rural poor, it seems clear that the migrant health problem is not an isolated one, but is but one sector of the rural poor health problem.

2. Under the first four proximate causes, solutions to those causes have been listed. The two major divisions of solutions would be environmental primary prevention (improve housing, improve quality of water supply, improve pesticide practices, etc.); and personal medical approaches, either preventive or therapeutic (detect diabetes, treat it, etc).

It is important to reemphasize here the impossibility of deciding with our present state of knowledge which services are the most cost-effective to provide, environmental preventive measures or personal medical services. We simply cannot say whether more diseases come about because of poor housing, or because of "natural" causes. Conventional wisdom tells us that the environmental hazards provoke disease in younger persons, and thus provide a bigger payoff when effected, but this is not certain as a statement of basic fact or value, especially when applying a discount rate to productive services rendered in the future. It is also said that certain small environmental approaches might cost little and have large positive effects—fixing the water supply, for instance. Housing is the biggest problem, however, and erecting good housing for migrants is not cheap. Furthermore, a great deal of usual medical practice is prevention, even while it is treatment. Control of a urinary tract infection in a young mother keeps her out of the hospital later on, and might even save her life, as well as making her a better mother and worker. Clearly, there is a role for both approaches, and to a certain extent they can be viewed as independent measures, although there is assuredly a degree of interconnection. So long as we cannot make specific statements of the prevalence and incidence of different diseases among the migrants, and so long as we cannot define quantitative causality patterns for each disease or disease cluster, we shall be unable to define the most cost-effective approaches to migrant health.

E. Summary

Figure 1-4 summarizes the causal pattern derived from the discussion in this chapter. Four "red herrings" have been cited that are most likely of but small import in causation of poor health among migrants; mobility leads to discontinuity of medical care, insufficient public health preventive services are delivered, health education is insufficient, and motivation to use health services is low. Most of the factors cited in figure 1-4 are applicable for the rural poor as well as the migrants, although often not to the same extent. We are unable to distinguish the cost-effectiveness of environmental prevention and the personal medical services approach for this population.

IV INTERVENTION POSSIBILITIES AND THE CRITERIA FOR JUDGMENT

Figure 1-4 should be read to make two major points: first, there are nine separate factors of greater or lesser importance that contribute to the causation of poor health for the migrants; second, the interconnections among these are manifold and very complicated. Clearly, a myriad of program possibilities could be developed to improve migrant health, each emphasizing one or another factor to a greater or lesser extent, and each using different approaches to the various factors. In this report we shall be evaluating only those solutions to the migrant health problem that have been suggested at one time or another by those involved in some capacity with the Migrant Health Program. Before examining them, however, it would be useful to examine briefly each of the nine factors to see the variety of approaches possible with each.

A. Varieties of Approach

Since *political-economic powerlessness* seems to lie behind most of the migrants' health problems ultimately–not to mention their non-health problems–we would naturally look there for a preferable solution. Realities being what they are (and the limits of this study what they are), this problem cannot be met head-on as the primary focus of a governmental health program. We must be content to keep this ultimate factor in mind, and indicate the effect proposed programs have on political-economic powerlessness as spillover.

Poverty can be alleviated by the provision of money. A direct grant of money would have this effect, as would provision of the opportunity to make money, as in training for a job. In a sense provision of any services is a payment in kind, and therefore is an antipoverty agent. Economics tells us that this latter alternative cannot be as Pareto efficient as the former method, unless the service is not obtainable on the open market. That medical care is often not purchasable in rural areas is the only economic defense for having a program specifically designed to alleviate migrant health at all.

In rating the various alternative approaches to solving the migrant health problem we shall be faced with the problem that all provide some sort of poverty alleviation, since they provide in-kind service or, in one case, direct cash. For the purpose of these rating only those approaches that seek to improve the migrants impoverishment directly, figuring that health will be improved as a consequence, shall be recognized.

Mobility can be compensated for by dealing with its effect. It is doubtful that the primary psychological problems engendered by mobility can be much ameliorated, for interruptions in the sense of community are inseparable from migrancy. Ineligibility for various welfare programs at the state and local levels because of migrancy could be changed, most likely by federal and state actions. Unfamiliarity with the local medical care system could be changed by providing an alternative system especially for migrants, or by establishing services designed to reach out to the migrant and insert him into the system. The lack of influence of the migrant with local governmental bodies resulting from absence in local elections could be compensated for by federal pressure and local legal advocacy. Self-help environmental efforts would seem to be beyond practicality so long as the migrant migrates at least upstream.

There are two basic approaches to alleviate *discrimination* in medical care. First, a separate system of care for the migrant could be established. The threat of a "separate but unequal" system could be countered by such steps as ensuring quality of care, employing staff from the same ethnic and economic group as the migrants, training the non-minority groups for sensitivity, etc.

Secondly, one could attempt to integrate the migrant into a system with others. "Others" could be either a poor non-migrant population where the same provisions for ensuring non-prejudice as above would apply—or the "others" could be a general group of medical care consumers, for instance, subscribers to a prepaid group practice. In this latter instance, the range of services would certainly not be prejudicial, as could happen in a separate arrangement, but internal discrimination would still be possible. Pechansky and Fox documented such an instance with a non-migrant minority group: "at the group with a large black clientele, blacks were referred significantly less than whites."[63] By the very nature of the setup it is difficult to employ minority group personnel, although not impossible; it would be very difficult to effect feedback control from the migrants.

A traditional general approach would be anti-discrimination community education. Some might be effective, but the record of such approaches to race relations is disappointing. Giving migrants job opportunities, and interfering with the poverty discrimination influence, might be more germane.

The problem of *increasing the capacity of the rural medical care delivery system* as a whole is beyond the scope of any program concerned primarily with the provision of medical care to migrants, although certain actions of the Migrant Health Program might have implications for the rural areas in general. In the local areas that the MHP might concentrate on, however, cognizance could be taken of the overall problem of capacity, and to the extent manpower were imported from outside instead of merely using local manpower, and to the extent that progressive forms of organization were stimulated in the area, it could be said that a particular solution sought to improve the state of health of migrants by increasing the medical care capacity in the areas in question.

Environmental improvement could be undertaken several ways. The growers could be pressured into doing a better job, as could local and state officials. Lobbying in the state capitols for better laws could take place. National standards could be set. The migrants could be organized into self-help action, mostly in home-base areas, or the MHP could undertake improvements directly. Local legal advocacy would be another approach. Union contracts with specific standards would be still another possibility.

Occupational hazards such as accidents, pesticide exposure, and highway accidents could be attacked in the same ways as environmental improvement.

Malnutrition could be attacked by direct distribution of foodstuffs, establishing automatic migrant eligibility for food stamps, and providing transportation for commodity distribution.

Medical care could be provided for the migrants in a great variety of ways. Mobile medical trailers could follow the migrant stream providing care. Medical personnel could be imported to migrant areas to give care in a traditional setting. Personnel could be organized into groups and care dispensed from that setting. Local providers could be utilized for all migrant care, or just for referral. Health departments could be asked to provide medical care. Other institutions, such as hospitals or medical schools, whether found locally or at a distance, could be asked to deliver care.

B. Judging Medical Care and Efficiency

In evaluating the proposed programs, special care must be taken in assessing the medical care factor, because of the great varieties of services that can be offered, and because judging them is a fairly abstruse process. In addition, we will want to give some estimate of the overall efficiency of the programs, even if we must judge roughly. We shall deal with these two issues in some detail now.

Clearly, some medical care is more valuable than other medical care. We must have standards to judge medical care provision, just as we must have standards to judge the provision of environmental health services, for example. But medical care is more difficult to judge than the other areas, although the others are not easy.

It is relatively easy for a layman to judge an environmental program, for instance. The water is contaminated or it isn't, there is epidemic diarrheal disease or there isn't. There are items that one would have difficulty deciding if they were desirable in themselves or as a means to something else—"adequate" space in a house, for instance, but in the main, evaluation of environmental efforts is rather straightforward.

Medical care, however, is difficult to evaluate in terms of end results—"longevity, activity, comfort, satisfaction, disease, achievement and resilience." [64] This assertion may sound suspiciously like a dodge by the medical profession, and to a certain extent it probably is. Nonetheless, the best experts in the field of medical care evaluation say that such an approach is difficult at best, and often misleading. [65]

End-result measures, or outputs, necessitate control groups which may be very difficult or impossible to find, and in addition need a long time for proper measurement—the ultimate results in different ways of treating an ulcer patient might need twenty or more years. Furthermore, defining the outputs is problematic. Is consumer acceptability an end or a means or both? To what extent is medical care consumption, and to what extent investment? Clearly, end-result measurements would be a very difficult way to evaluate the different kinds of care one might propose to give the migrant population.

It is more appropriate to judge medical care by the common standards utilized by professionals in the field, that is, by process (or input) measures. There are four key criteria for assessing medical care delivery: (1) technical quality of the services provided, (2) comprehensiveness of services provided, (3) accessibility of services provided, and (4) acceptability of services provided. Each item is important, and each enhances the net effect more in the presence of the others than it would alone.

1. By technical quality of services provided we mean, first of all, the degree to which the treatments and advice provided conform to the best medical opinion for each episode of illness. Continuity of care is included as a parameter. Whereas end-result measures would be of necessity measure whether or not the current medical opinion were effective (by measuring whether patients got better or not), we take a more restricted view, and assume that most of what the best physicians recommended is indeed helpful. A second aspect of quality consists of the efforts taken by purveyors of care to ensure good quality maintenance by periodic chart reviews, patient conferences, and other measures.

Quality of services is obviously important; the tough question is where to draw the line. It is unlikely that every service should be Mayo Clinic quality; it is even more unlikely that every service should be what current medical opinion would class as poor. A good rule of thumb for our purposes would seem to be that the common diseases that are important to diagnose and treat must be handled properly. In addition, important but less common diseases must be recognized and proper handling be provided for. The term "handled properly" means according to best medical opinion. An example would be that a first urinary tract infection in a female would require history, physical examination, urinalysis, culture of the urine, and antibiotic treatment on the first visit, with a follow-up visit after discontinuation of the therapy for urinalysis and culture once again. Less than satisfactory quality would be, at the extreme, diagnosis by history of urinary tract symptoms and therapy on the spot without follow-up.

We admittedly do not know the cost-effectiveness ratios involved between the above two alternatives. Perhaps we would save enough money by cutting down service to the latter inferior level to do more good for more people *in toto*. In general, however, it is probably fair to say that most bad medicine is practised not to increase the cost-effectiveness ratio, but for other reasons such as poor training, insufficient equipment, or poor administration. Since no one has even tried to construct a scheme that would increase overall welfare by decreasing the quality of individual services, it would be irresponsible for any program to set out to provide inferior care willfully on a large population. We can say, then, that no program should accept quality of care less than each physician has been trained to give under normal circumstances.

2. Comprehensive services means the full range of outreach, preventive, diagnostic, therapeutic, and rehabilitative care tied together in an integrated package, not just existing separately and diffusely in a community.

The necessity of such an array arises when one analyzes the services appropriate to various patients at various stages of their diseases. It becomes even more important when one realizes that not handling a patient at the proper time with the proper services means handling the patient at another time with different services, and this would prove undoubtedly more expensive and less efficient for both the facility and the patient.

To cite examples of variable needs: all children need measles immunizations, or many will experience many days of morbidity (that will also involve the mother), and some will die. Ear infections are common but there is often little one can do to prevent them; the important thing is to treat them when they crop up, and keep following them up to prevent hearing loss, which might well occur and permanently injure the child educationally, and prevent him from progressing. Urinary tract infections can hardly be prevented, although some health education is no doubt beneficial; once again the important thing is to treat them before pyelonephritis and chronic kidney damage ensue, perhaps necessitating hospitalization, morbidity, and mortality. Trauma can be prevented somewhat, but treatment and rehabilitation are exceedingly important; treatment without rehabilitation would be very inefficient. Another common malady is hypertension; here, early case finding and preventive supervision with pressure-lowering drugs and dietary and social advice would be the approaches of choice.

The above varieties of common diseases are cited to emphasize that comprehensiveness entails a balance of components. Rather than being a luxury, comprehensiveness of services is the only sensible approach to the variety of diseases to which man is heir. Some diseases cannot be prevented, at least most of the time (hypertension); some cannot be treated (measles encephalitis); many need rehabilitation after treatment for the patient to be productive (broken hip).

Some diseases, such as urinary tract infection, if not treated at an early stage, will progress and wind up costing everyone more.

There are no data assessing cost-effectiveness of which services to provide in which order; it is only clear that all services are applicable for some diseases at some point, and all services must therefore be provided, although we cannot say what ratio they should bear to one another in size. We can say, however, that it makes sense to provide generalized services that can adapt to the variable patients. Specialized clinics for common diseases are not particularly cost-efficient in themselves, and are clearly unable to take care of the broad range of illnesses exhibited by populations. To cover the whole population categorically disease by disease would require innumerable clinics, which would be clearly inefficient for all involved.

3. Accessibility of services defines the ease a patient experiences in obtaining services when he desires them. Easy accessibility increases utilization of services and in most populations increases the appropriateness of care. This is because of the importance of executing preventive procedures that have little immediate obvious payoff,[66] as well as treating diseases early. Convenience to the patient in time and place of services increases accessibility.

Other means of increasing accessibility are to expedite enrollment and eligibility-ascertaining procedures, to establish a mixed appointment and drop-in schedule, and to provide transportation services. All but the last involve mostly administrative arrangements, and little change in costs.

4. Acceptability of services to the patient population is desirable in itself, as with any consumer good or service. In addition, acceptability increases quality and appropriateness of care in the same way as does accessibility. The "placebo effect" of patient-physician relations is enhanced by acceptability. Finally, patient cooperation with the physician and compliance with his recommendations, often deficient,[67] is improved with more acceptable care.

No formula to produce acceptable care exists. In the past, city hospitals and other institutions serving the poor usually produced largely unacceptable care; the private sector, on the other hand, satisfied its patients for the most part. More recently, it seems that the two sectors have tended to come closer to each other in this dimension. While private practitioners have become overloaded with cases and have stopped making house calls, public medicine has made strides forward with Neighborhood Health Centers and other innovations. Typical steps taken by the Neighborhood Health Centers to improve acceptability have been employing personnel deriving from the same social group as the patients, designing facilities to ensure privacy and dignity, and attempting to receive continuous feedback from patients on the services offered. Such criteria as these must be used in assessing acceptability of services.

It is not clear how one reconciles the need to provide the above ingredients in some degree in all services with the need to make a small budget spread as far as possible. In other words, one must have some idea of the relative worth of each component as that worth changes as more and more of the component is added. In addition, the components are synergistic. Take, for example, quality of services and accessibility. It would mean little to have high quality services that were inaccessible, or accessible services of low quality. Rather, each component provides more by virtue of the other's being present.

At any point in a project, then, the greatest payoff might be gained by investing in one or another of these four aspects. Each component is necessary, but not sufficient for proper delivery of medical care. In trying to make money stretch as far as possible, a balance in each individual project must be respected.

Each proposed plan must be rated for efficiency. Efficiency in this context means not the overall effectiveness of the strategy proposed, but rather the cost-effectiveness ratio of the specific components envisioned, and the ratio of services delivered to administrative overhead.

Once again, medical care deserves special mention in this regard. Most productive processes are characterized by decreasing unit costs as the firm gradually builds up its scale, but decreasing returns to scale after a certain point is passed. The medical care process seems to fit this description. Practically, what does this mean? A physician must have an X-ray machine and technician available to practice medicine properly. Not having one available would seriously undermine the quality and quantity of the physician's production. To keep an X-ray machine fully employed, one needs several physicians supplying it. (There are even more economies to be had in using a hospital's X-ray, but there are countervailing diseconomies one must consider involving location, bureaucracy, etc.) One could say the same about the laboratory and electrocardiograph machine. Even assuming the modest ratios of two clinic nurses, one public health nurse, and three aides per physician, an absolutely minimal project with three physicians, one lab technician, one X-ray technician, one receptionist, three clerical staff, and one administrator, has a personnel list of twenty-eight. Few would claim the unit cost curve had yet started to increase, and the personnel budget at $12,000 average per person would be $336,000.

It certainly seems as though once a county were to be chosen for a migrant health project it would make sense to build up the scale of the operation so that it could serve all the eligibles in the area, since economies of scale would be accrued all along the way. At the far extreme of expansion, however, it might well be that diseconomies would take their toll. In rural areas there is an extra cost for each more remote area one chooses to serve; expansions to the periphery would entail ever decreasing returns. Furthermore, the most eager to be served show up for service first; as the degree of recalcitrance grows, so does the cost of expanding the operation. Other diseconomies must accrue as well. Minimization of these diseconomies would be effected by choosing the most congested counties as primary targets.

Vague as the figures involved are, it should be clear that in a local project a budget of $500,000 annually would be on the descending portion of the unit cost curve.

Finally, to be complete we should consider one other aspect of any program that might be devised to solve the migrant health problem. That is, to what extent does the program contribute to the solution of problems of the migrants other than health, such as education, jobs, exit from the migrant stream, and so on. This accounts for the final column of evaluation criterion, criterion, "spillover effects."

C. Summary

Figure 1-4 presents nine different precursors of poor health of migrants, any one or more of which (with the exception of political-economic powerlessness) could be attacked in a program to improve the health of migrants, each in several ways. It will be enough in most cases to simply note to what extent a program attacks each category. In the case of medical care, however, the issue is rather more complex, and it will be helpful to describe the type of medical care provided in terms of four criteria: quality, comprehensiveness, accessibility, and acceptability. Overall efficiency will be another point of judgment, and this, too, will hinge primarily on the medical care arrangements, although other factors could weigh in as well. The final point of description will be for spillover effects, according to non-health benefits supplied to the migrants.

Our check list of criteria, then, will consist of the following items: (1) poverty alleviation, (2) mobility alleviation, (3) discrimination alleviation, (4) increase of capacity of rural medical care delivery system, (5) environmental improvement, (6) occupational hazard alleviation, (7) malnutrition alleviation, (8) medical care provision, (8a) type of medical care provided, (9) efficiency of operation, and (10) "spillover" effects.

V SUMMARY OF CHAPTER 1

I. Description of the migrants

Migrant workers and their families possibly number as many as one million persons, are mostly young, black or Chicano, have low educational achievements, bad housing and environment, and very low incomes. Their state of health is poor, and receipt of health services low. Excluded from coverage under basic labor laws in the 1930s, the migrants were recognized in the Migrant Health Program of 1962, and subsequently in several Great Society programs. They are still excluded de facto from many potentially helpful programs, as well as the basic labor laws.

II. Problems of rural health care

Rural area public sector health services consist of environmental sanitation and marginal personal services; the poor are not generally well served by this sector. The private sector delivers the bulk of personal medical services, cannot meet all the demands placed on it, and suffers from both manpower and organizational insufficiencies. Active steps are necessary to solve these problems, but of the five most important approaches in the past, none has been very successful. New federal manpower programs and efforts to promote Health Maintenance Organizations will have important implications for future solutions.

III. The problem of migrant health—causation

Figure 1-4 summarizes the causal pattern of the poor health of migrants derived from the discussion in this chapter. Most of the factors apply to the rural poor in general as well as the migrants, although often not to the same extent. The cost-effectiveness of environmental prevention and personal medical services for this population cannot be distinguished.

IV. Intervention possibilities and the criteria for judgment

Figure 1-4 presents nine different precursors of poor health of migrants, any one or more of which could be attacked in a program to improve the health of migrants, and each of which could be attacked in several different ways. In describing the various approaches it will usually suffice to note the extent to which a program will attack each category. Medical care is rather more complex than the other categories, so we shall add another point of judgment on that issue, and assess the appropriateness of the type of care according to quality, comprehensiveness, accessibility, and acceptability. Overall efficiency will be another point of judgment, and this too will hinge primarily on the medical care arrangements. The final point of description will be for "spill-over" effects, assessing non-health benefits supplied to the migrants.

Chapter Two

The Classical Migrant Health Program

This chapter traces how the federal government responded to the health needs of the migrants from 1962, when the Migrant Health Program (MHP) legislation was passed, to 1970; this is the "classical" period of the MHP. In 1970 the MHP underwent some upheaval, and projects that deviated from the "classical" pattern were funded. Although these aberrent programs have survived, the "classical" program was not at all destroyed, but rather continues on. Evaluating the "classical" program is therefore of more than historical interest.

The primary sources of information utilized in this chapter are described in Appendix D.

I LEGISLATION

The Migrant Health Act, section 310 of the Public Health Service Law, (see Appendix A) was originally passed in 1962, and the first funds appropriated in 1963. Two types of projects were authorized by the legislation: (1) family health service clinics, and (2) special projects to improve health conditions. Most of the projects funded have fallen in the first category. Two types of special projects have been supported: a few "sanitation-only" projects, and numerous projects undertaken by state health departments with the primary purpose of supplying consultation to local projects.

The law specifies that grantees to operate these projects may be "public and other nonprofit agencies, institutions, and organizations," and does not specify that such grants need to be passed through the state health departments. The legislative history does not indicate that some cooperation with the state health departments was expected, but that the discretion of the federal program administrators was to be relied upon.

The dollar authorization for the Program began at $3 million, was at $51 million in Fiscal Year 1970, $20 million in FY 1971, $25 million in FY

1972 and $30 million in FY 1973 and FY 1974. The corresponding appropriations were: $15 million in FY 1970 and 1971, $17.95 million for FY 1972, $23.75 million for FY 1973, and effectively $23.75 million in FY 1974 (actually, in FY 1974 $25 million was appropriated with a 5 percent discretionary cut available to the administration). (See fig. 2-1). The latter appropriation represents less than $25 per migrant,[a] as contrasted with about $400 per person average expenditure for medical care in the general population currently (including indirect expenditures).

Significant amendments occurred in 1965 when the Program was enabled to pay for hospitalization for its patients, and in 1970, when the Program was enabled "to provide health services to persons (and their families) who perform seasonal agricultural services similar to the services performed by domestic agricultural migratory workers if the Secretary finds that the provision of health services under this sentence will contribute to the improvement of the health conditions of such migratory workers and their families." The 1970 amendments also called for involvement of the consumer population and "others in the community knowledge about such needs" in planning and implementing the projects.

II PROGRAM OPERATIONS

Figures 2-2 through 2-13 and tables 2-1 through 2-8 indicate the manner in which the Migrant Health Program administrators chose to distribute their funds. The data for these graphs come from the sources indicated in Appendix D. That we have had to make use of such methods of obtaining figures for these straightforward graphs and charts, and that such graphs and charts were not readily preparable from program data, let alone already prepared by the program, speaks for the level of evaluation and data collection that the program achieved. This point will arise again.

A. Size of Grants

The median and modal *grant size* coincide at $50,000. The mean grant is worth $61,000. Figure 2-2 shows that many more small grants are funded than rather larger ones, but even the latter are less than $280,000, which is not a large amount compared to most federally funded comprehensive medical care projects. If we place total dollars spent instead of number of grants on the ordinate, as in figure 2-3, the emphasis is more spread out within this small spectrum. Figure 2-4 shows that 53 percent of the program's grant funds go for grants worth less than $100,000 individually.

[a]The Control Systems Research study, referenced in the notes to Chapter 1, showed 70 percent of migrant families spent less than $100 per year on various aspects of medical care.

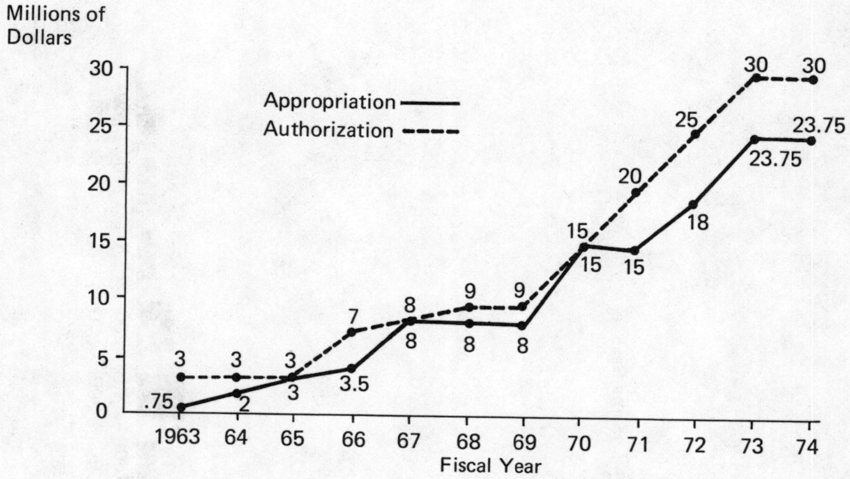

Figure 2-1. Migrant Health Program Funding.

B. Project Location

Figures 2-2 and 2-3 show that "upstream" projects tend to dominate in the lower valued grant categories, and home-base grants in the more richly funded. Figure 2-5 shows that many more small grants than large grants were given to upstream areas, and the same relation holds, but less strikingly, for home-base areas. The second comparison to be drawn from figure 2-5 examines total dollar value rather than number of grants. We see here that rather small grants predominate upstream, but in the home base, funds are divided rather equally between larger and smaller projects. Figure 2-4 shows us that overall 57 percent of the funds go to upstream areas, 43 percent to home base. Table 2-1 displays the same picture by percentage of each size of project home base or upstream.

C. Project Sponsorship

Project sponsorship is predominatly by the health department at every level of project, as table 2-2 shows. Overall, 67 percent of the projects are sponsored by health departments, 16 percent by local voluntary agencies (usually a "migrant council" or church group), 9 percent by local governmental bodies (other than the health department, usually county commissioners), and 4 percent by medical societies. Figure 2-6 shows that analysis by total of funds instead of number of projects makes the health department share appear even larger. Figure 2-3 shows that as the project size grows, the share of the health departments tends to become greater. This point is also made by figure 2-7. The breakdown of project sponsors by project and location (table 2-3) is instructive.

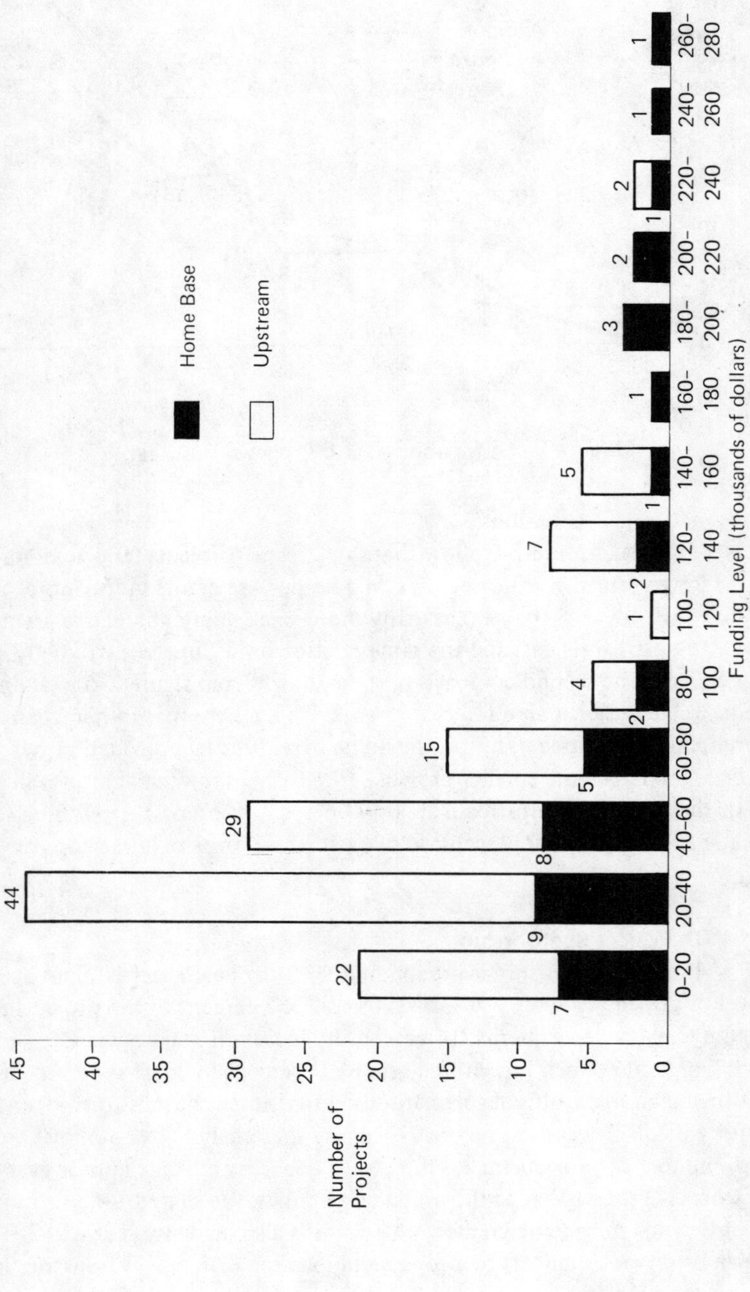

Figure 2–2. *Size of Grant per Project* FY 1970 (State Level and New Grants Excluded).

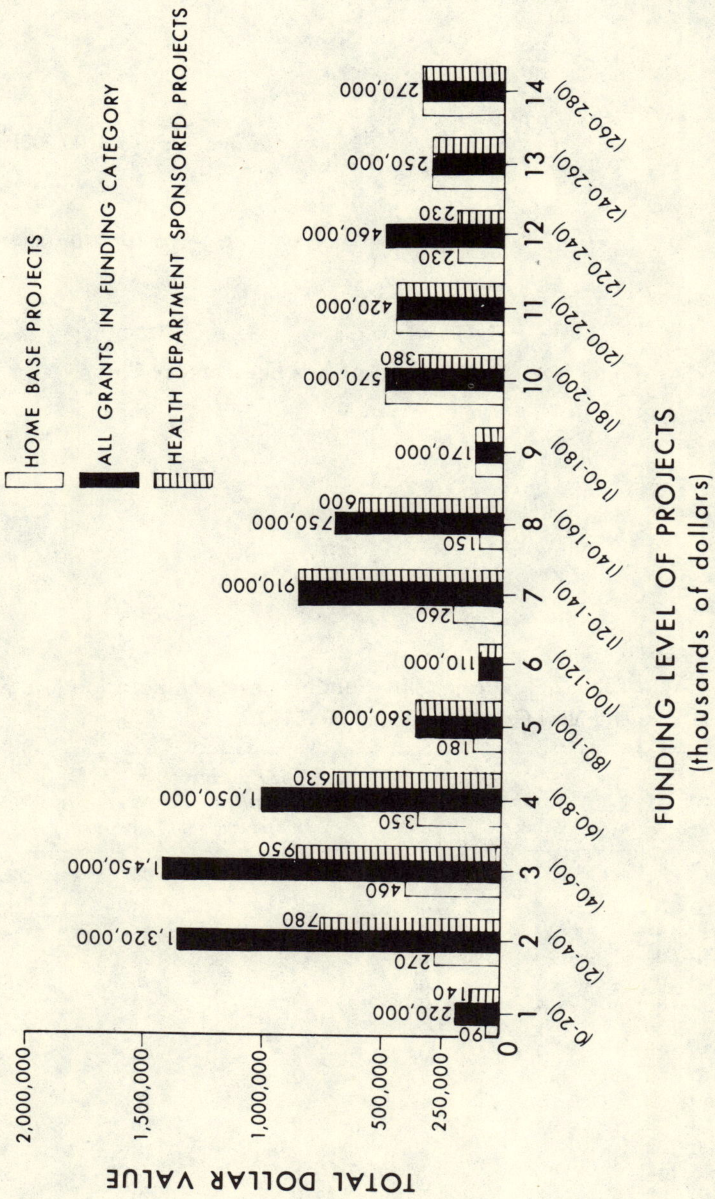

Figure 2–3. *Total Amount of Dollars Granted, by Size of Grant* (State Level and New Grants Excluded). FY 1970.

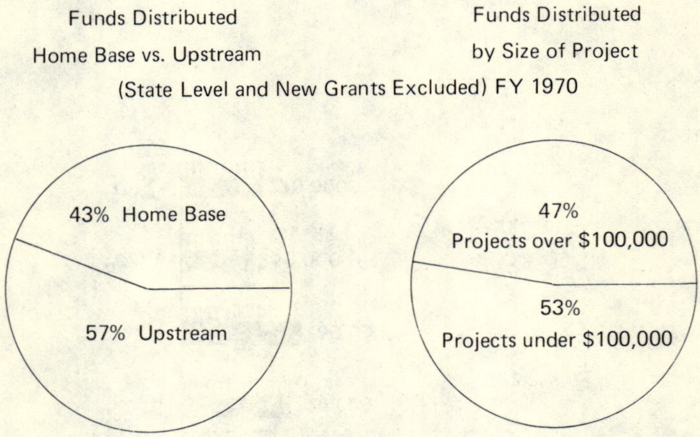

Figure 2-4. Projects by Funding Level and Location.

Table 2-1. Projects by Funding Level and Location (State Level and New Grants Excluded) FY 1970

Funding Category	*Number of Projects*	*Number of Homebase*	*% of Projects in this Row Homebase*	*Number of Upstream*	*% of Projects in This Row Upstream*
All	137	43	31%	94	69%
1. 0–20	22	7	32%	15	68%
2. 20–40	44	9	21%	35	79%
3. 40–60	29	8	28%	21	72%
4. 60–80	15	5	33%	10	67%
5. 80–100	4	2	50%	2	50%
6. 100–120	1			1	100%
7. 120–140	7	2	29%	5	71%
8. 140–160	5	1	20%	4	80%
9. 160–180	1	1		0	0%
10. 180–200	3	3	100%	0	0%
11. 200–220	2	2	100%	0	0%
12. 220–240	2	1	50%	1	50%
13. 240–260	1	1	100%	0	0%
14. 260–280	1	1	100%	0	0%

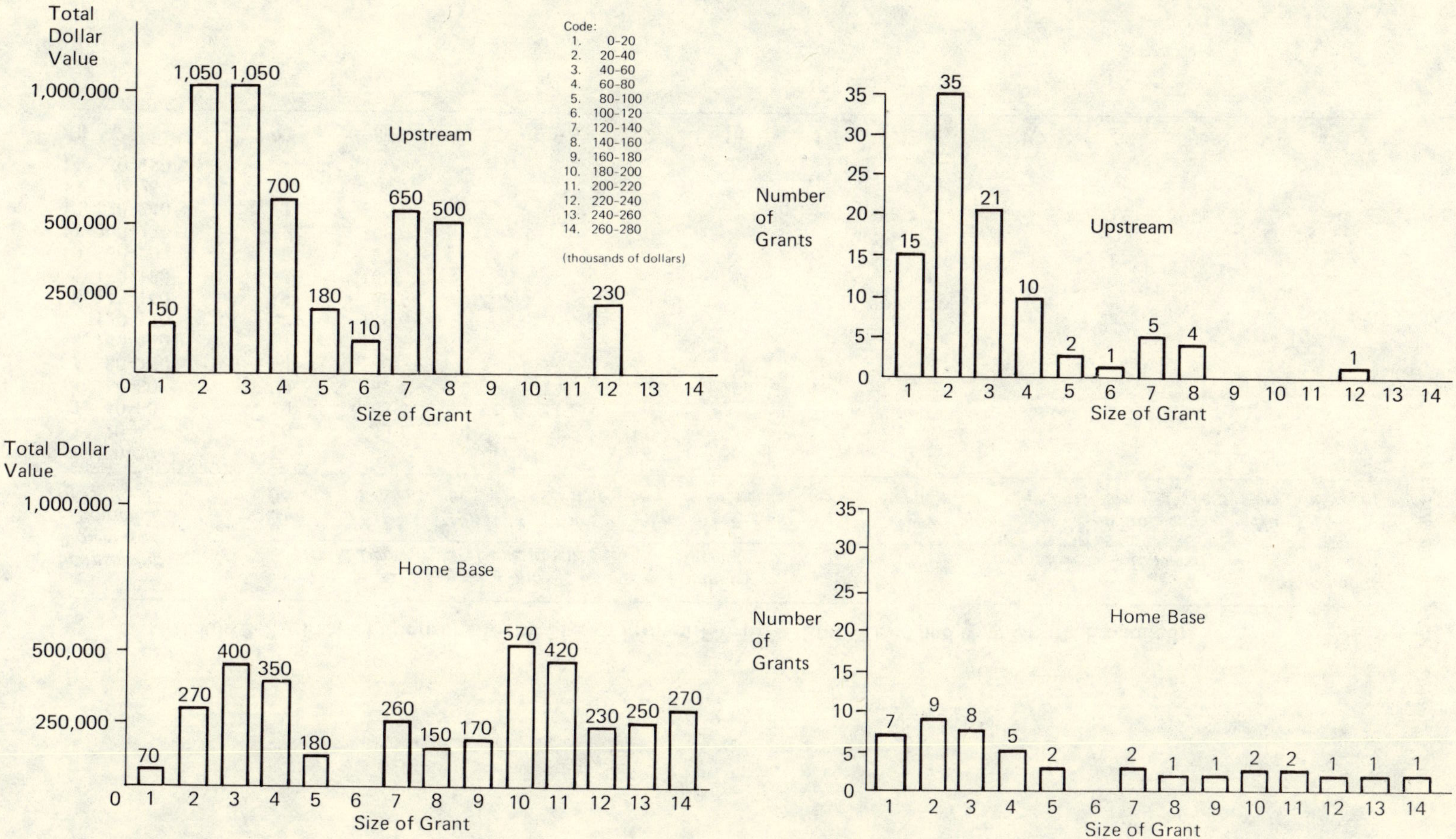

Figure 2-5. *Location, Number of Grants, Size of Grant, and Total Money Awarded.* FY 1970 (State Level and New Grants Excluded).

Table 2-2. Project Sponsorship, by Size of Project FY 1970 (State Level and New Grants Excluded)

Sponsorship Project Size (Thousands of Dollars)	Health Dept.		County Government		Voluntary Agency		Medical Society		Hospital		University		State Labor Commission	
	Number	Percent	Number	Percent	Number	Percent	Number	Percent	Number	Percent	Number	Percent	Number	Percent
1. 0–20	14	64%			8	36%								
2. 20–40	26	59%	4	9%	11	25%	1	2%	1	2%			1	2%
3. 40–60	19	65%	7	24%			2	7%	1	3%				
4. 60–80	9	60%	2	13%	3	20%	1	7%						
5. 80–100	4	100%												
6. 100–120	1	100%												
7. 120–140	7	100%												
8. 140–160	4	80%					1	20%						
9. 160–180	1	100%												
10. 180–200	2	67%									1	33%		
11. 200–220	2	100%												
12. 220–240	1	50%									1	50%		
13. 240–260	1	100%												
14. 260–280	1	100%												
All	92	67%	13	9%	22	16%	5	4%	2	1%	2	1%	1	1%

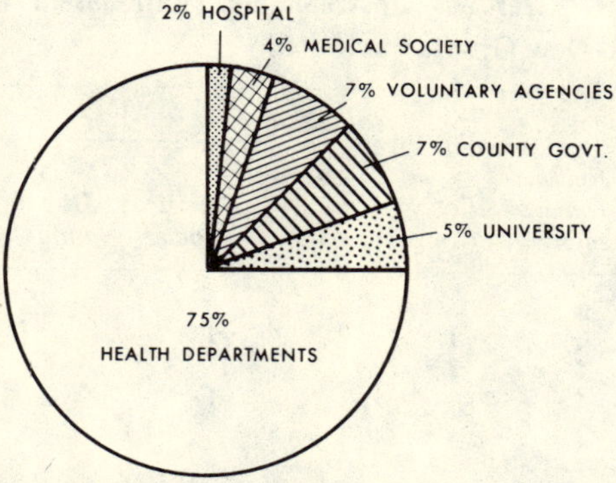

Figure 2-6. *Funds Distribution, by Sponsorship* FY 1970 (State Level and New Grants Excluded)

The major differences in the home-base and upstream totals occur in the health department and voluntary agency columns: home-base health departments, 77 percent, and voluntary agencies, 5 percent; upstream health departments, 63 percent, and voluntary agencies, 21 percent. The bottom row of the home-base and upstream figures are almost identical. Both areas place primary reliance upon health departments; upstream areas differ from home base by utilizing voluntary agencies one-fifth of the time.

D. Project Size and Migrant Concentrations

The significant but relatively mild correlation between project size and number of migrants in the area to be served is charted in figure 2-8.

Most projects cover a rather small portion of the eligible population in the area. Examination of the sample of twenty-five projects taken by the

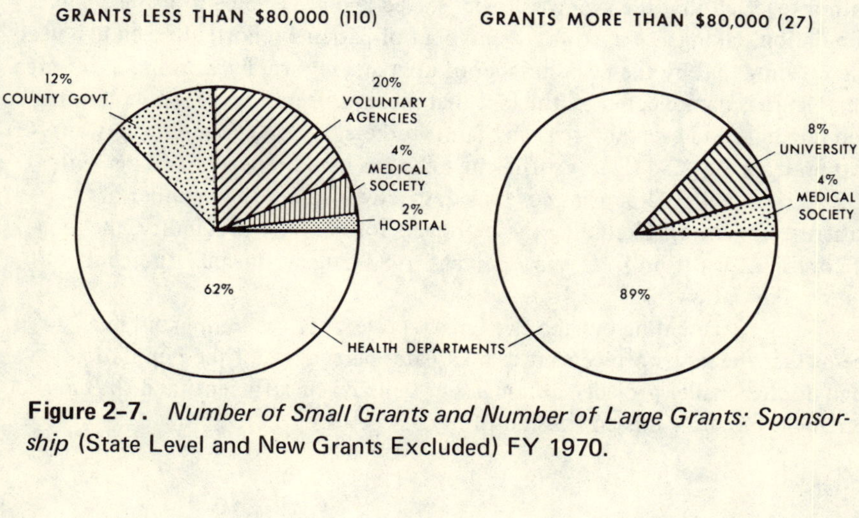

Figure 2-7. *Number of Small Grants and Number of Large Grants: Sponsorship* (State Level and New Grants Excluded) FY 1970.

Table 2-3. Grantees, Upstream and Homebase, FY 1970 (State Level and New Grants Excluded)

	Homebase						
Project Size	*Health Department*	*Local Govt.*	*Voluntary Agency*	*Medical Society*	*Hospital*	*University*	
1. (0–20)	6		1				
2. (20–40)	6	1	1	1			
3. (40–60)	4	3			1		
4. (60–80)	4			1			
5. (80–100)	2						
6. (100–120)	7						
7. (120–140)	2						
8. (140–160)	1						
9. (160–180)	1						
10. (180–200)	2					1	
11. (200–220)	2						
12. (220–240)	1						
13. (240–260)	1						
14. (260–280)	1						
Totals	33	4	2	2	1	1	43 tot.
Totals, by %	77%	9%	5%	5%	2%	2%	100%
Totals, omitting Vol. Agency	33	4	2	2	1	1	41 tot.
Totals, by % omitting Vol. Agency	80%	10%	5%	5%	2%	2%	99%

author revealed that the average project served about 31 percent of the eligible population, taking as a measure the number of patients reportedly seen in a year, and dividing that by the peak number of migrants reportedly working in the area. This figure is complicated by the fact that most projects openly report treating non-migrants and even non-seasonal farm workers. In fact, three of the twenty-two projects that had figures sufficient to be evaluated reported 118 percent, 132 percent, and 332 percent coverage respectively (counting number of patients, not visits)! Excluding these projects for non-interpretability, the range of coverage for the projects was 7 percent to 83 percent, mean 31 percent, standard deviation 23.

Segmenting out the five largest projects of the sample in table 2–4, it seems that the larger projects cover no greater percentage of the population than do the smaller projects, although our sample is insufficient (and the data too unreliable) to draw this conclusion firmly.

	Upstream							
Project Size	*Health Department*	*Local Govt.*	*Voluntary Agency*	*Medical Society*	*Hospital*	*University*	*State Labor Comm.*	
1	8		7					
2	20	3	10		1		1	
3	15	4		2				
4	5	2	3					
5	2							
6	1							
7	5							
8	3			1				
9								
10								
11								
12						1		
13								
14								
Totals	59	9	20	3	1	1	1	94 tot.
Totals, by %	63%	10%	21%	3%	1%	1%	1%	100%
Totals omitting Vol. Agency	59	9		3	1	1	1	74 tot.
Totals, by % omitting Vol. Agency	80%	12%		4%	1%	1%	1%	99%

E. Coverage of States

As of 1969, thirty-seven states had projects. The state health department consulting projects were twenty-five in number, and received a total of $903,135 in grant funds. Including both this last figure and the amount of money granted for service projects either directly to the state, or through the state to a local health department (the predominant practice in Florida, California, and Oregon) state health departments received a total of $4,565,134 in grants. Fourteen of these states got more than $100,000; the California State Health Department got more than $1 million; the Florida State Board of Health nearly $600,000; and the Oregon State Health Department nearly $500,000.

F. Stability Through Time

We have some evidence that the above patterns were as true in 1964 as in 1969. The American Public Health Association study of December 30,

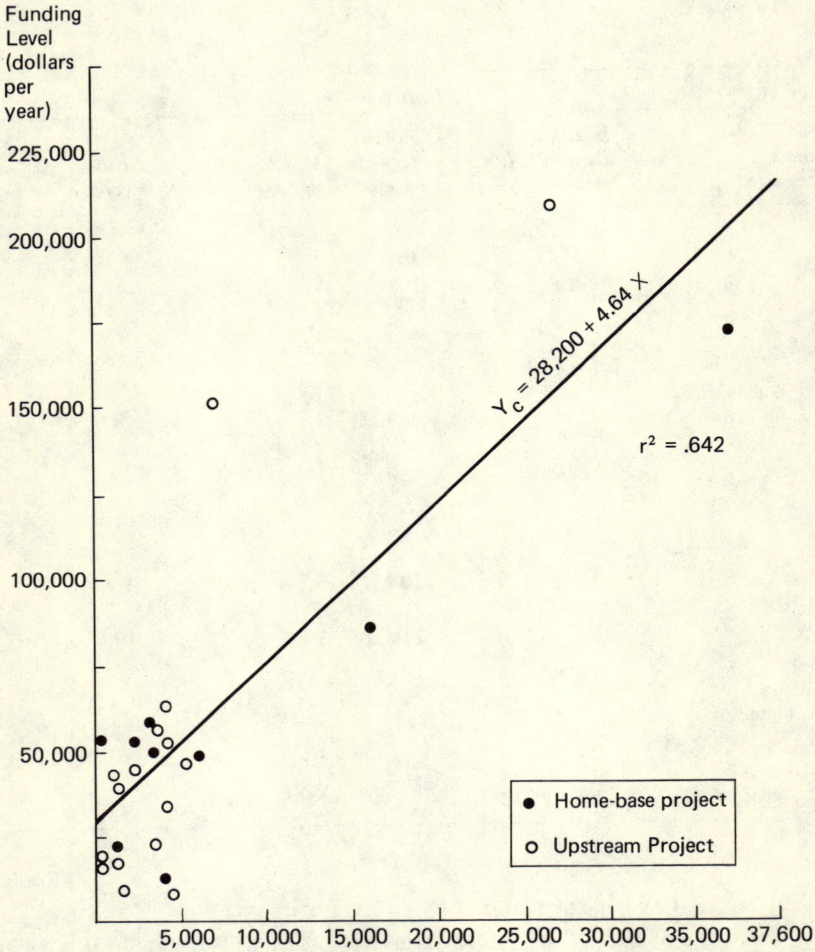

Figure 2-8. Correlation Between Peak Migrant Population in County, and Project Funding (25 Sample Projects).

1964 lists a total of forty-five projects funded from $2.5 million total grant funds available, for a mean of $53,000 per grant. Of the forty-five projects, only eleven were located in home-base states—Florida, Arizona, Texas, and California—while thirty-four were upstream. Forty of the forty-five projects show health department sponsorship. Despite the increase in funding and passage of six years, then, it seems the pattern of funding changed little.

Not only was the pattern maintained, but so were a great many of the very same projects, as reference to figure 2-9 will confirm. Although it is not clear how many and which projects have been dropped from the program, by all accounts and by the evidence of figure 2-9, discontinued projects have been

Table 2-4. Population Coverage of Five Largest Projects from Sample

Project Size (annual budget)	*Percentage of Migrant Population in Area Served*
$210,000	28%
172,000	10%
151,000	29%
85,000	17%
61,000	17%

very few in number. The average project age after eight years of the program was 4.8 years. (For these figures the county projects in Florida and Oregon had to be excluded, since individual data were not available.)

G. Strategy Behind Patterns

The Program policies would seem then to have been quite stable through the years. It is quite difficult, however, to reconstruct the rationale for these policies. Unfortunately, the Program seems to be devoid of strategy

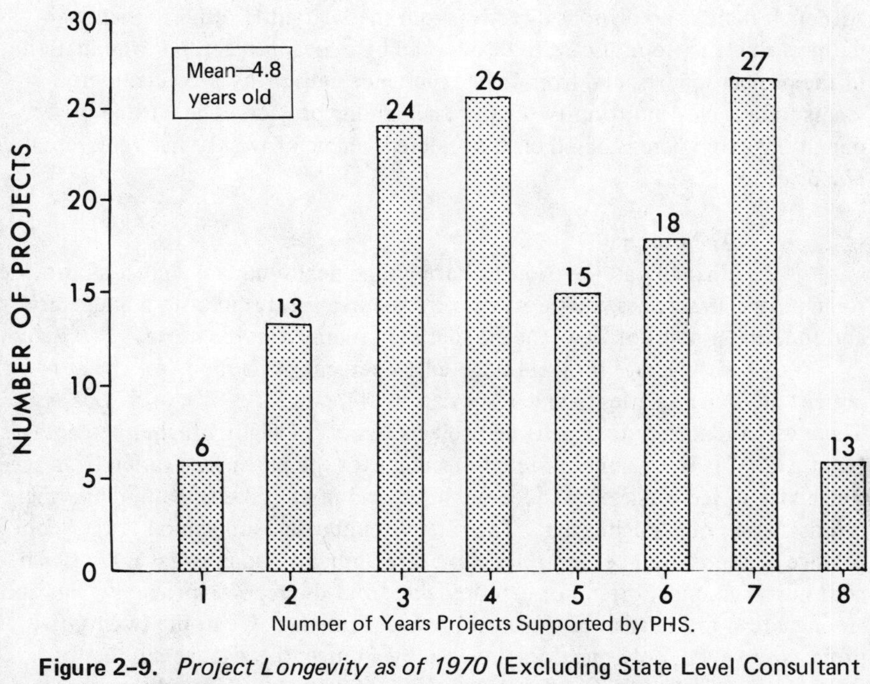

Figure 2-9. *Project Longevity as of 1970* (Excluding State Level Consultant Projects and New Projects FY 70; also Excluding County Level Projects in Florida and Oregon).

documents. Furthermore, interviews with Program personnel who were making these policies tend to be lacking in detail.

We shall restrain ourselves from speculating upon the reasoning of the administrators, and simply accept as data the end result of what they did. They faced a difficult task of trying to decide what kind of health care services to give to a population of about a million mobile persons with only $3, and later $8, per person to work with.

H. Summary

The majority of grants and the greater part of the grant money in FY 1969 were for *small size* rather than large size grants, more grants and more money went to *upstream* rather than home-base areas, and the great majority of grants and total funds went to state and local *health departments.* Furthermore, there seems to be no relationship among the areas. Both the general patterns of money distribution and the specific projects funded tended to be quite stable over time. There are no positive data to suggest the conscious strategy of the administrators.

III PROJECT ORGANIZATION AND OPERATIONS

Although there is no obvious directive from the Migrant Health Program mandating a single pattern of care to be adopted by a local project, on examination of the project reports, and from field experience with many projects, there seems to be a clear uniformity of approach among projects. The outline of operations given here is based on the selected sample of twenty-five representative projects.

A. Personnel

Virtually all the projects have public health nurses, almost all provide some physician services, and most employ a sanitarian. From both a budgetary and functional point of view, the emphasis is generally on the nurse.

The average project budgeted 14 percent of its funds for the outpatient physician salaries (standard deviation .09, range .02–37), or $7,648. There was a tendency for upstream projects to budget slightly higher percentages (see fig. 2–10). The manner of reimbursement for the physicians varied from fee-for-service to fee-per-session to fee-per-hour, and in one case a health department physician was on straight salary. The rate of reimbursement generally was "competitive"–$15 or $20 per hour per clinic session being about average. Physician continuity was most often not determinable from the reports; probably, rotation among a few physicians was the most prevalent practice. Of all the twenty-five projects surveyed, only one does not employ a nurse; the average number of nurses in a project is 2.5 (see fig. 2–11). If $7,500 were considered the average salary for a nurse, the average project of the sample spent $18,750 on nurses.

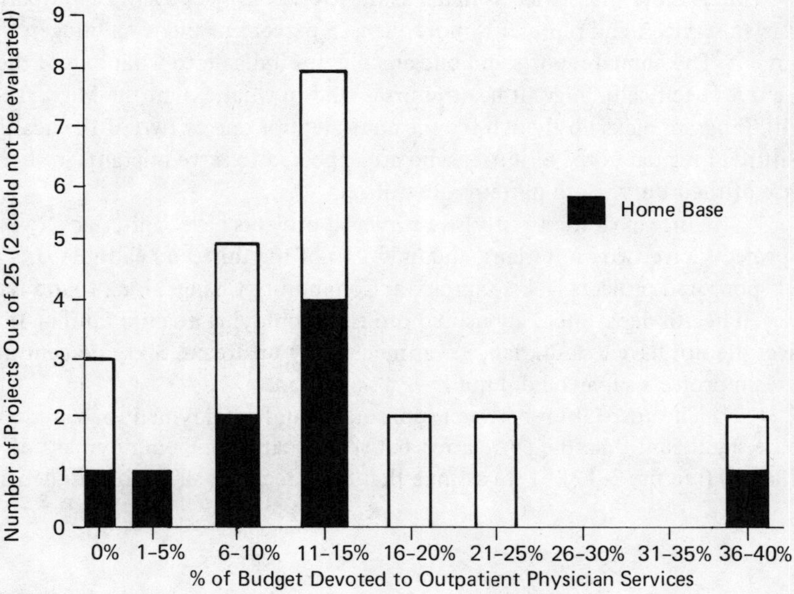

Figure 2-10. *Percentage of Budget Devoted to Outpatient Physician Services* (Sample of 25 Projects).

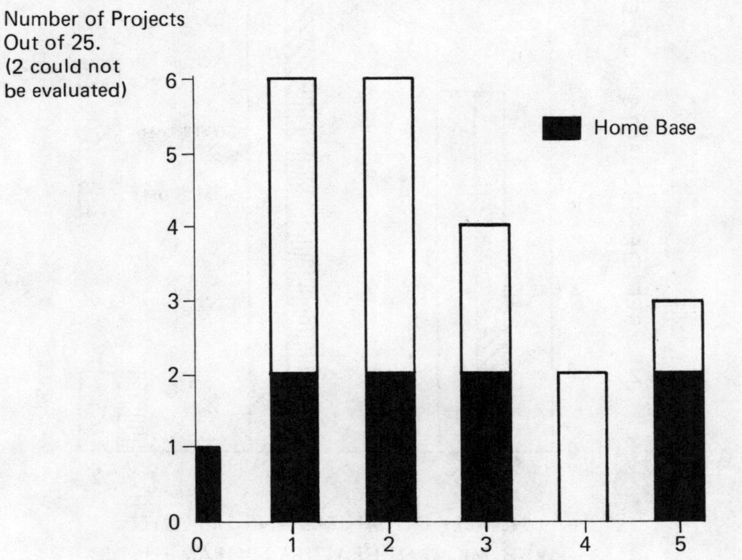

Figure 2-11. Number of Nurses per Project Paid with Migrant Health Program Money (Sample of 25 Projects).

This figure is more than twice as much as the average project spent on outpatient physician services, and represents more than 25 percent of the total budget allotment. The annual reports and budgets did not indicate to what extent the nurses are specifically migrant health nurses, and to what extent the Migrant Health Program picks up the tab for the equivalent of one or two of the health department regular corps of nurses who are expected to serve migrants in the course of their duty. Both patterns are utilized.

Fifteen of the twenty-five surveyed projects have sanitarians; two of the projects have two sanitarians, and only two of the thirteen health department sponsored projects lack a sanitarian. Community Change, Inc., found ten of eleven health department sponsored projects employing a sanitarian.[1] If a project did not have a sanitarian, it was most likely upstream. Sixty percent of upstream projects surveyed did not have a sanitarian.

The correlation between sponsorship and employment of sanitarians is more significant than the correlation between location and employment of sanitarians (see fig. 2-12). If we assume that 85 percent of all the health depart-

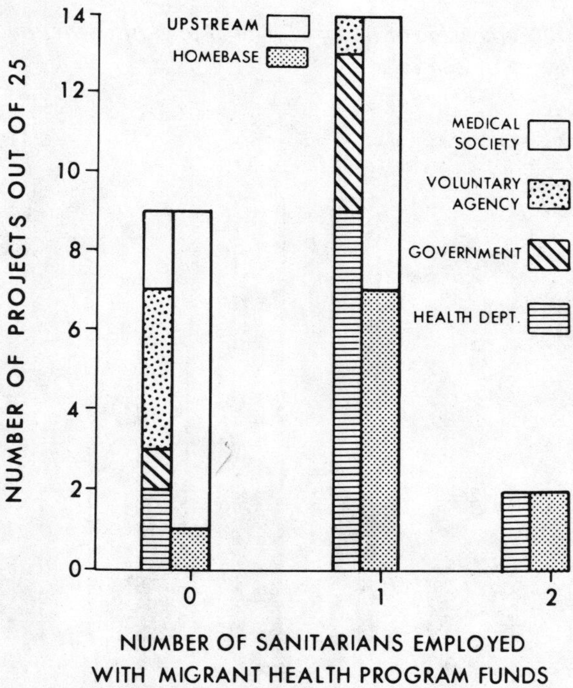

Figure 2-12. Sanitarians Employed by Projects Paid with Migrant Health Program Funds (Sample of 25 Projects).

ment sponsored projects have a sanitarian, and 33 percent of all the non-health department sponsored projects, since health departments sponsored two-thirds of all the projects, we can calculate that probably about two-thirds of all projects have sanitarians. Taking all the projects from our sample which employed at least one sanitarian (fifteen projects), we find their average expenditure on outpatient physicians to be $7,740. In other words, these projects spend about as much on sanitarians as they do on physicians.

Only seven of the twenty-five projects employed aides of any kind. Experience with the program indicates that few of these aides come from migrant families or even from the same ethnic or economic group as the migrants. Employment of local residents well-disposed toward the migrants is more common. No aide is used in an innovative manner, and career development for the aides is not considered.

B. Medical Care Delivery

Twenty of twenty-five projects surveyed offered periodic general medical clinics, most designed to serve a single area once or at most twice a week. This finding is consonant with the findings of the APHA report, which found clinics meeting once or twice a week, and offering much less than comprehensive services. [2] Thirteen of the projects offered referral services to local physicians. 80 percent of the projects offer general clinics, 52 percent offer fee for service referral. The results of the survey are charted on table 2-5. Of the five projects offering fee for service referral only, four are in Texas.

The thirteen health department sponsored projects had a clinic 94 percent of the time (table 2-6).

It could not be determined from the reports to what extent the typical health department categorical clinics (VD, TB, well-baby, etc.) were utilized. There were, however, frequent references in the annual report narratives to the fact that the health department categorical clinics were open to migrants; to what extent Migrant Health Program money supported such an activity was unclear. The Community Change evaluation found ten of eleven health department sponsored projects offering categories clinics. [3] It could also not be determined how many of the clinics were night clinics and how many at convenient locations; from experience, we can estimate that most home-base projects have daytime clinics, often at the health department offices, and that the

Table 2-5. Physician Services Organization, By Project

	Upstream	*Home-base*	*Total*
Clinic only	5 (33%)	7 (70%)	12 (48%)
Referral only	3 (20%)	2 (20%)	5 (20%)
Clinic and referral	7 (47%)	1 (10%)	8 (32%)
Total	15 (100%)	10 (100%)	25 (100%)

Table 2-6. Physician Services Organization in Health Department Sponsored Projects

Clinic only	9 (79%)
Referral only	2 (15%)
Clinic and referral	2 (15%)
Total	13 (99%)

upstream clinics often meet at night, not infrequently at makeshift facilities near the migrant camps.

With few exceptions the clinics in which the physicians work have no ability to supply simple laboratory, X-ray, or electrocardiographic analyses on site (see table 2-7).

The evidence strongly indicates that the physicians face tremendous loads in their clinic services, and must spend only small amounts of time with each patient accordingly. The impact of this burden is made more obstrusive by the fact that many of the clinics operate at night, when the physicians have already done a full day's work and are tired. Although the annual project reports give information insufficient for a systematic appraisal on this question, the following indications are very suggestive:

1. "Health for the Harvesters," a California Farm Workers Health Service publication, says that a physician may be called upon to see seventy to eighty patients a night in seven hours time.[4]
2. Such a project reports as do make mention of patient loads most often tell of situations similar to that found in California.
3. The field experiences of several Migrant Health Program workers confirm the above reports.
4. Two physicians from the central office of the Migrant Health Program spoke with many project physicians throughout the country in an effort to formu-

Table 2-7. Laboratory and X-ray Facilities of 25 Selected Projects

	Home Base Projects	*Upstream Projects*	*All Projects*
Laboratory on-site	1 (10%)	1 (7%)	2 (8%)
Laboratory not on-site	6 (60%)	7 (47%)	13 (52%)
Laboratory uncertain from report	3 (30%)	7 (47%)	10 (40%)
Total	10 (100%)	15 (101%)	25 (100%)
X-ray on site	0 (0%)	0 (0%)	0 (0%)
X-ray not on site	4 (40%)	10 (67%)	14 (56%)
X-ray uncertain from report	6 (60%)	5 (33%)	11 (44%)
Total	10 (100%)	15 (100%)	25 (100%)

late medical care guidelines in 1969. They found that an almost constant complaint was insufficient time available to evaluate a patient properly (insufficient laboratory, X-ray, and electrocardiographic clinic capabilities was another constant complaint).

5. The evidence that twice as much project money is devoted to nurses as to physicians indicates that the patient-generating, case-finding activities are overemphasized as compared to the direct patient care activities. This deduction can be made because nurses come more cheaply than doctors, and can probably generate more patients per dollar than a physician can process per dollar. In other words, if a physician is paid an average of $20 per hour, and a nurse $4 per hour, and twice as much money is devoted to nurses as doctors, each project budgets ten nurse hours to each physician hour. Although nurses spend some of this time in patient processing rather than patient generating, it seems clear that projects budget much more case-finding than case-processing, and the result is logically an overloading of clinics.

The physician, then, most often can spend very little time with each patient.

We cannot tell with any precision from the annual report narratives what the balance might be between clinic and public health duties (home visits, follow up, case-finding, health education, etc.) for the nurse, but since the clinics meet but once or twice a week usually, and the nurses are full-time employees, we can infer that the major part of their duties is public health nursing. Of the functions within the rubric of public health nursing, it is most probable that the concentration of nurses is on case-finding, health education, and triage (separating the well, the sick, and the sicker), rather than on delivery of physician initiated procedures to patients in the clinics or the field. Close coordination between the nurse and the physician is necessary for the latter activity to proceed, and we have good evidence that such coordination is at best very difficult in the migrant health projects. Both annual report narratives and site visit assessments indicate that the following factors, which would inhibit such coordination, are commonly present: frequent rotation of medical personnel at the clinics; the practice of rotating clinic nurses, and having the traveling nurses and clinic nurses neither identical nor in close communication with one another; overburden of clinic physician loads; lack of record keeping and planning as a consequence of clinic overburden; practice of frequent referrals to physicians in a setting physically distinct from the clinics. It is doubly unfortunate that the nurses must concentrate on functions not directly connected to physician services, for not only are the latter services frequently more productive than the former, non-directly physician related ones, but moreover, the nurses face additional barriers of language and cultural gaps from the patients. These gaps make the productivity from health education and case-finding even less than it would be otherwise.

C. Environmental Services

The annual reports give evidence insufficient to define clearly the usual functions of the sanitarians. Generally, it seems, snaitarians act under the state and local responsibility given to health departments to enforce the sanitation laws. Their actions could consist mainly of camp and housing inspections, sewage disposal inspection, water inspection, food inspection of restaurants, etc. The laws ensure that the enforcers have neither the mandate nor the funds at their disposal to effect such corrections as might be necessary themselves; they can merely cite violations as they find them. The process of obtaining corrections is a difficult one, although the figures given by the annual reports show a high degree of compliance generally, and as such are quite at variance with field experience of migrants, federal officials, and other investigators. Generally, the owner of the facilities in question is told of the violations, and attempts are made to persuade him to change. In the case of housing, it is often considered a success if the housing is declared unfit for human habitation. As with the early experience in urban renewal, little effort is spent on locating or providing better housing for the individuals involved. The essentially impossible situation of the county sanitarians is detailed in a study made by the California Rural Legal Assistance.[5]

Sanitarians have not extended their activities to problems of field sanitation, where workers are generally forced to urinate and defecate in the fields, nor to pesticide poisoning, nor to occupational accident prevention.

Community Change, Inc., in their 1971 evaluation of the Migrant Health Program done for the Department of Health, Education and Welfare, documents some of the practical problems with the MHP's environmental efforts:

> The visits to projects sponsored by state and local public health departments suggest that frequently the grant funds support the ongoing activities of the department without significantly increasing services to migrants. Of the ten projects paying for sanitarians (all with health department sponsorship), nine appear to be using them for substantial non-migrant work. For example:
> –Charleston, South Carolina, has a 6-month salary for a sanitarian in an area with 6 weeks of migrants and not one labor camp which meets minimum federal standards;
> –Kern County, California, pays part of a sanitarian's support, although labor camp inspection is a state function in California;
> –Collier County, Florida, has two sanitarians covering all general sanitation (septic tanks, motels, restaurants, etc.) in most of the county, yet entirely paid by project funds;
> –Seminole County, Florida, has a full-time sanitarian, yet there is only one labor camp in the county. The one time the camp has been used in the past two years, the sanitarian did not inspect it;

–Laredo/Webb, Texas, has two sanitarians actually doing social case work and certifying the eligibility of migrants for other programs;
–Zapata, Texas, has two full-time sanitation positions and no labor camps.[6]

Although the Community Change study concentrates on the essential duplicity of the projects, the California Rural Legal Assistance point remains the central one: with current laws and current political and organizational structure at the county level, the job of sanitarian cannot be successfully filled.

D. Health Education Services

The Migrant Health Program administrators have placed a great deal of emphasis on health education in such documents as have been issued, and their consultations to projects and the project review process have generally emphasized health education. Few professional health educators, however, seem to have been employed by the local projects. The annual reports do indicate that the project personnel, most particularly of course the nurses and sanitarians, participate heavily in health education activities. Talks to meetings, slide shows, and personal consultations in the homes and camps seem to be common. Since both project organization and local circumstances deny nurses and sanitarians the opportunity to act directly, they are naturally drawn in the direction of health education.

E. Inpatient Care

Since the 1965 amendment to the law, projects have been able to pay for hospital and physician inpatient expenses of migrants. Thirteen of the twenty-five projects the author surveyed had such components. The average percentage of the budget expended for inpatient services in these projects is 29 percent, range 10–55 percent, standard deviation .15. Figure 2–13 indicates that over one-half of the projects with hospitalization spent between 11 and 30 percent of their budgets on such expenses, but that 15 percent spent over 50 percent of their budgets in that manner (see table 2–8).

F. Consumer Orientation

None of the projects surveyed gave evidence of having an advisory board of consumers of care (the year of reporting was before passage of the Mondale amendment requiring establishment of such boards). Moreover, none gave any evidence of the reaction of patients to the services provided, any complaints or patient problems with the services, or any corrections that had been made. Employment policies generally excluded the hiring of persons with a "migrant-type" background. In site visits generally project personnel responded to such inquiries by pointing to their patient loads, although the absence of alternative sources of medical care nullifies the validity of their argument.

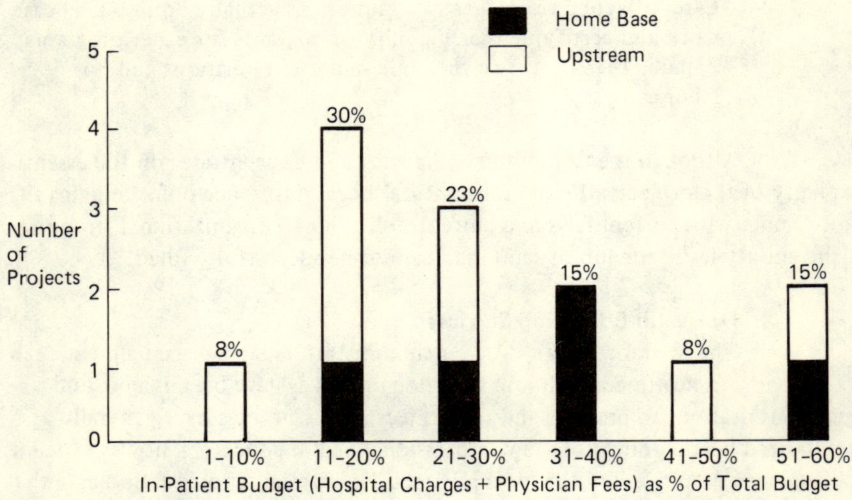

Note—% Figures at Top of Bar Refer to Proportion of Projects from Our Sample Falling into that Category (e.g. 8% of Projects Budget 1-10% of Their Funds for Inpatient Services.)
—Graph Includes Only Projects with Inpatient Care as Line Item from Sample of 25 Projects.

Figure 2-13. Percentage of Budget Devoted to Inpatient Care by Project.

G. Summary

The MHP projects of the "classical" period bear a strong similarity to one another. In the category of personnel, nursing services are heavily emphasized, more than twice as much money being spent on them as on physicians, despite the nurses' considerably lower pay rates. Sanitarians are also emphasized, as much being spent on their services as on physicians'. Aides are not at all extensively used, and not in innovative ways when they are. On the average, 25 percent of a project's budget is spent on nurses, 14 percent on physicians.

Medical care is delivered in 80 percent of the projects through general medical clinics and in 52 percent through fee-for-service referrals. The usual health department categorical clinics are usually supplied when the project sponsor is a health department. Most home-base projects have daytime clinics held at the health department offices, most upstream projects have nighttime clinics held at makeshift sites near the camps. The clinics almost never have laboratory, X-ray, or electrocardiographic capabilities on site, and the physicians spend very little time with each patient. There are too many nurses in proportion to the number of physicians; the nurses for the most part perform the public health functions of case-finding, health education, and triage, but can perform and follow up physician-initiated activities to only a small extent, thus decreasing their productivity significantly.

Environmental services are limited to the traditional health depart-

Table 2-8. Percentage of Budget Devoted to Inpatient Care as Related to Percentage of Budget Devoted to Outpatient Physician—Sample of 25 Projects

Project #	*% Budget Devoted to Inpatient Care*	*% Budget Devoted to Outpatient Physician*	*Inpatient % Outpatient%*	*Home Base*
1	0	0		x
2	0	0		
3	0	6		x
4	0	7		
5	0	13		x
6	0	13		x
7	0	13		
8	0	17		
9	0	18		
10	0	37		
11	10	8	1.3	
12	14	6	2.3	
13	14	11	1.3	
14	19	11	1.7	
15	20	11	1.8	x
16	21	14	1.5	
17	22	12	1.8	x
18	29	21	1.4	
19	34	37	0.9	x
20	35	2	17.5	x
21	49	23	2.1	
22	52	0	∞	
23	55	9	6.1	x

(2 projects had figures insufficient for analysis.)

ment inspection duties, which the health departments are legally expected to perform on their own. Political obstacles to successful fulfillment of environmental functions are pronounced, and in practice these functions indeed seem to be performed poorly by the projects. There is no evidence of efforts with field sanitation, pesticide control, or occupational hazard protection. Health education services are dispensed by both sanitarians and nurses.

Over half the projects reviewed had inpatient care components, spending on the average 29 percent of their budgets on it; the amount spent on inpatient care was usually one to two times as much as that spent on outpatient physician care. No project gave evidence of formal or informal channels for receipt of consumer feedback, let alone compliance with consumer wishes.

IV PROGRAM EVALUATION

Two evaluations shall be considered in this section: the program's evaluation of itself, and our own evaluation of the program.

A. Self-Evaluation

We can deal with the program's evaluation of itself very shortly and simply, for there has been extremely little of it.

In presentations to Congress, the program has generally cited two kinds of statistics that bear upon performance of the program: (1) numbers of various services provided, and (2) number of counties in which such services are offered. For example, in the December 1967 publication by the Senate Subcommittee on Migratory Labor, "Migrant Health Program, Current Operations and Additional Needs," a chart is supplied that summarizes the typical data supplied by the program, in its fullest extent (see Appendix E). Two points are to be made relating to this chart. First, there is good reason to question the accuracy of the figures. Reliable informants among program officials state that not only are project data submitted with cavalier disregard for actuality in many projects, but moreover, there is really no compilation made of the separate project to get the program figures. The author has not attempted to verify these figures by actually doing such a compilation. Suffice it to say neither he nor anyone he spoke to in the program is aware of any person who actually did the figuring, nor of any charts or documents internal to the program from which such figures were taken for the official figures given to Congress. There is never any explanation given in any of the Migrant Health Program prepared documents of the sources of data.

The second point to be made about the data presentation is that, even if the figures are accurate and reliable, they would indicate very little about the value or impact of the program. The number of medical visits, dental visits or nursing visits tells nothing about what kind of visits they were (immunization? screening? general medical clinic?), whether they resulted in a valuable outcome or not, what the quality of the services was, etc. The same can be said about sanitation inspections.

Similarly, indicating how many counties have and have not migrant health projects (Appendix E, from the same December 1967 report) and citing the statistic of "number (of migrants) in project areas at some time during year" gives a false impression that these counties and persons are "covered" for migrant health services. In fact, projects and counties are of very different sizes, and adequate coverage of health needs is rarely if ever effected by any of the migrant health projects (see statistics of section D above) in any area. The figures as presented give equal weight to a project of $50,000 and one of $500,000, if each were to be located in a county with 10,000 migrants at some time of the year. Clearly, such a statistic is misleading.

Of course, statistical displays to Congress are usually not intended to constitute an unbiased and objective critique of a program's efforts. We cite these presentations here only because there is very little else we can find that might be taken to represent some effort at program evaluation. The discouraging aspect of the congressional presentations is that not only are the figures unreliable and presented to give an illusory impression, but the figures are not even capable of being reworked under different evaluative constructs to give some useful information.

Internally, the program simply does not evaluate either the overall impact of its efforts nor even the relative success of various individual projects in a serious and systematic way. The author could find no evidence of any program review statistics, or even narrative, compiled for the use of anyone, with the sole exception of an effort to computerize and classify hospital admissions (still incomplete after several years). An illustrative incident is the following: In 1970 the Rural Housing Alliance requested from the Migrant Health Program a state-by-state breakdown of expenditures on sanitation by the Migrant Health Program. Simple as this request was, the MHP was forced to respond that it had no such data available on a state-by-state basis, and indeed could give only an estimate for the entire program expenditures (the sanitarian consultant of the MHP said that the Program has generally used the figure 8–10% of funds for sanitation, although he emphasized that this was no more than an estimate)! Such an incident is indicative; the veracity of figures supplied by the MHP must be doubted.

Lack of evaluation is evident at the simpler level of the individual projects as well. The projects have been required to submit annual reports listing various statistics, such as total number of visits, distribution of medical conditions seen, sanitation inspections completed, etc. The impression is widely held that the projects do not take their reporting duties seriously, and thus simply make up figures that would sound reasonable and rather flattering; some project directors have openly admitted as much. Other projects leave many of the reporting spaces blank, impunitively. Their behavior is understandable—the figures would not aid the projects themselves in self-evaluation and direction, and little is often made by the MHP administrators.

The central administrators treat the figures with great distrust, virtually ignoring them. Were the figures accurate, something could be made of them. Such data as average cost per patient visit, average percentage of patients diagnosed with various diseases, ratio of nursing to physician costs, average grant per person eligible in area could be computed. Certainly a much better system of reporting could be developed, but at least something would be possible with the present system. Not only are the present statistics not analyzed, but no general compilation of statistics is produced to enable others to make calculations. The figures lie deep in the project reports (themselves often not so easy to track down), and are effectively buried. Eschewing "hard" data, the administrators rely on the "general impressions" of the regional representatives and others who have visited the project. Since the annual reporting form does not require an organizational description, even a qualitative analysis on this subject is impossible.

Information on the projects, in sum, is insufficient to support objective analysis.

B. Evaluation by Criteria

In Chapter 1, part IV, we took the outline of causes for ill health among migrants and noted how intervention might take place at various points to effect an improvement in the health of migrants. Checking the "classical" Migrant Health Program against these points will put the intent of the Program into perspective.

(The rating scale from 0 to ++++ below denotes for points 1 to 8 and point 10 the extent to which the solution devotes its energies and resources toward that problem. For point 8a, the rating denotes a judgment of the appropriateness of the medical approach according to medical care criteria previously discussed. Point 9 takes account of the mix of factors selected for attack, as far as that is possible, as well as the individual approaches suggested.)

1. Poverty Alleviation (0).
   This route of intervention was only undertaken to the extent that health services were delivered for free, and thus provided in-kind income. This approach does not constitute what we would define as an attack on poverty. (For the purposes of this analysis, as mentioned in Chapter 1, section IV, we assume that any program designed to improve the health of migrants to some extent affects their poverty, by supplying income in-kind, and by remedying conditions that prevent migrants from working. Under the present rubric of poverty alleviation, we are interested in programs that seek to alleviate poverty primarily, and calculate that an improvement in financial status would lead to an improvement in health status).
2. Mobility Alleviation (++).
   This route of intervention is adopted somewhat by the program, in that specific efforts are often made to make the migrant aware of the existence of the local migrant health project, to make services accessible specifically for him by offering evening clinics in camps, and to provide for some referral of patients within the stream. No efforts to curtail the mobility itself, or to make the migrants eligible for social and medical welfare programs are made.
3. Discrimination Alleviation (+).
   This route of intervention is utilized somewhat, in that services that are separate from those supplied to non-migrants are supplied. Steps such as

hiring minority personnel, or establishing patient feedback channels, are not taken. Some small effort is also undertaken under the rubric of "health education" to educate the surrounding community to the problems and assets of the migrants, in an attempt to improve prejudiced attitudes.

4. Increasing Rural Medical Care Capacity (0).
   This route of intervention is not utilized. Rather, personnel that are already situated in the area are used, and no efforts are made to attract other personnel. Furthermore, little effort is made to increase physician productivity by reorganizing service arrangements.
5. Environmental Improvement (+).
   This route of intervention is firmly adopted by the program conceptually. About two-thirds of the classical projects have at least one sanitarian employed. The orientation of the environmental approaches, however, leads us to doubt strongly that their effects could be extensive (see p. 64).
6. Occupational Hazard Alleviation (0).
   No documents, directives, or practices of the program point to this approach as an objective.
7. Malnutrition Alleviation (0).
   The author is aware of one project with a nutrition aide and a few that mention nutrition as a point for health education, but all in all, this approach is not much emphasized by the Program.
8. Medical Care Provision (+++).
   Direct provision of medical care is the major thrust of the program. although diluted by health education, sanitation, and other endeavors.

8a. Type of Medical Care Provided (0).
   Although the official rhetoric of the program called for comprehensive care with maximum feasible continuity, the reality of the service patterns as sketched in the previous section is such that services are better described as concentrating on episodic, symptomatic care in clinics, and in rather low-productive "health department" type prevention and nurse-intensive pursuits. It is worthwhile at this point establishing rather firmly that the services rendered by "classical" MHP projects are of low quality.

Although the data collected by the program are inadequate, inaccurate, and essentially uncompiled, an impression of the quality of medical care delivered by the program can still be obtained. We shall make use of "structural criteria," which provide concrete and relatively incontrovertible evidence of input capability. Such criteria serve the purpose of identifying situations where it is impossible to give good care, by virtue of the inherent limitations of organization, facilities, or personnel. That is, these criteria separate out those situations that *must* be deficient from those that may not be.

For adequate quality medical care to be delivered, a properly qualified physician (or other appropriate personnel) must see the patient for an appropriate amount of time in the proper facility with proper equipment on hand. Elementary laboratory and radiological capability must be available on site for care to be of adequate quality. The diagnosis of such important and common maladies as anemia, urinary tract infection, pneumonia, and fractured bones depends on that capability. It is accepted doctrine in primary medical care administration that the capability must be on site. What happens when they are not is most often similar to what a site investigation found in Maricopa County, Arizona, where one of the larger projects is situated:

> Laboratory services, as they exist now, are supposedly provided by the County Hospital. Urinalyses are sent without refrigeration in 110° weather to the hospital, and reports supposedly come back to the clinic within seven days. If blood chemistries are needed, the patient must transport himself to the County Hospital and present himself to the intern on duty with a note from Dr. _____. If the intern sees fit, the test is drawn. In practice, these procedures are so cumbersome and time consuming that, (a) results rarely are sent back to the clinics on time, *if at all*, (b) the blood tests are seldom drawn, because the patient has neither the time nor transportation, and the intern is not always inclined to cooperate, and (c) Dr. _____ has all but given up ordering these tests for reasons (a) and (b).[7]

The APHA 1964 analysis found "Lab facilities were conspicuously absent in project clinics".[8] The twenty-five project survey made by the author confirmed that the same situation still held in 1969 (see table 2–7).

Another structural criterion is time spent per patient. Even the world's best physician cannot do a good job if he is able to see each patient for only five minutes or less, provided that patient is not a routine follow-up patient, as virtually all migrant health patients are not. Under very rushed condition (with a language-cultural gap to boot) the physician can do no more than make an informed guess as to what might ail the patient, and treat him accordingly. Although some patients are lucky enough to be helped by this process, many are treated improperly, and many are given spurious reassurance by having been seen and evaluated by a physician. Evidence that grossly insufficient time per patient is available to migrant health clinic physicians is strong (see p. 62). The quality of the medical care rendered to patients is a casualty to this congestion.

Structural analysis can also be used to judge elements of quality that are non-technical in nature. Such an element would be degree of dignity with which the patient is treated. Undeniably, almost none of the projects' physical facilities approach the quality of the average private practitioner's office. Most have no wall separation of patients being examined, only curtains. Furthermore, most have no appointment system, but instead simply process patients on a first come, first served basis, and accept the resulting congestion and long patient waiting periods. The language and cultural gulf between staff and patients only exacerbates this unfortunate lack of dignity.

The medical services offered by the "classical" MHP projects are thus seriously deficient in quality and acceptability. Comprehensiveness of services is also obviously lacking. Of the four prime aspects of care, then, only accessibility seems to be provided by the "classical" MHP.

9. Efficiency (0).
The efficiency of the "classical" MHP could not be high. First, let us examine the program level. The large disbursements for state level consulting grants ($900,000 in FY 1969) plus disbursements for federal management (800,000 in FY 1969) indicate 19 percent non-service expenditures just to start with, not including individual project overhead.

Secondly, it is difficult to make a case for good efficiency when the quality of the major final product delivered, medical care, has been found to be quite poor.

Thirdly, the applicability of the minor final product delivered, environmental law enforcement, has been shown to be low, and in addition has been shown to be the responsibility of other duly authorized public authorities already.

Fourthly, the component balance in the medical care sector is poor. The projects have been shown to have relatively extensive nursing components, and relatively small primary care physician components. No one can say exactly what the ratio should be between these two components, but it is apparent that maximum efficiency is gained by having the physician-nurse relationship close enough so that the nurse can perform physician-extension type activities in the field. For such teamwork to develop, the physician must be doing more than simply spending a night a week seeing a patient every five minutes. Furthermore, recall that the average project had 2.5 nurses working full time, and one physician at a clinic once a week, or twice a week at most. Although a nurse might take a longer time per patient, it is exceedingly unlikely that her 100 hours (2.5 X 40 = 100) are producing the same number of patients as are the physician's five. The components are clearly out of proportion. (Alternatively, one could figure as we did in "Project Organization and Operations" that ten times as much time is spent by nurses as by doctors. Both ratios seem far out of line.) This whole argument, of course, also assumes the physician should be allowed much more time per patient, so an evaluation can be performed that is worthwhile for the nurse to follow-up. The argument is made *a fortiori* with this requirement.

The large hospitalization component of some projects provides another instance of component imbalance. In these projects "short-circuiting" occurs, with patients being shuttled from an active nursing program to an inpatient status without being intercepted by the weak outpatient care component.

Fifthly, the projects make virtually no use of aides. The many functions that are appropriate for them are probably performed by the nurse, which is of course inefficient.

Sixthly, the "classical" MHP projects are clearly of far too small a size to be taking advantage of economics of scale, as explained previously (see Chapter 1, Part IV, B., p. 37ff. The deficiency would seem to be of one order of magnitude (a factor of ten). Nor is there significant evidence of sharing resources with other endeavors and thus taking advantage of economies of scale to that limited extent. Attempts to share resources located away from the site of services are usually in vain. Health departments holding clinics in their own offices rarely have the kind of equipment necessary, and encounter other inefficiencies from the patients' point of view. (An illustration would come from Orange County, Florida, where the clinic location forced black migrants to enter the white section of town at night, an obvious inefficiency from their point of view.)

For all these reasons, then, the "classical" MHP should be considered quite inefficient.

10. Spillover (0).
The effect of the classical MHP on other goals of migrants—more jobs, retraining, education, etc.—is minimal. The projects are organized and run by professionals using almost exclusively non-migrant purveyors of care. The project goals are narrowly confined to health.

The "classical" MHP concentrated its efforts, then, on cause numbers 2, 5, and 8. Although many arguments can be offered for and against these choices, it is more profitable here to concentrate on the particular methods used in each category. The medical care effort must be vitiated by the type of medical care chosen, as rated under criterion 8a, and as detailed in the previous section of this chapter. The approach to environmental improvement is also clearly rather barren theoretically as well as practically. The value of attacking the problem of mobility by increasing access to poor health services must be considered low. Finally, the overall low efficiency of the program, and the low efficiency of the projects that derives from the faulty individual approaches, combine to give a picture of a "classical" MHP that delivered poor services with much waste.

In addition, we should recall the wasted motion of emphasizing two "red herring" causes. One is health education, which the official rhetoric of the MHP emphasized, and which was apparently reflected in many of the chores of the project nurses and sanitarians. The second is inter-project continuity. Even as late as FY 1970 a project was funded for about $150,000 to promote continuity along the Eastern stream. We have argued above that inter-project continuity becomes a significant priority item much further along in time, if things go right.

The difficulty of trying to devise a program to serve one million mobile persons with health services on a budget as low as the MHP's should not be underestimated. Nonetheless, it seems fair to observe that the route of intervention elected was at best unimaginative, and the manner in which it was effected was clearly inappropriate.

The following is a causal profile summary:

(1)	(2)	(3)	(4)	(5)	(6)	(7)	(8)	(8a)	(9)	(10)
0	++	+	0	+	0	0	+++	0	0	0

V SUMMARY OF CHAPTER 2

I. Legislation

The MHP legislation authorizes family health services clinics and special projects, with any public or non-profit private agency as sponsor. The original authorization was for $3 million a year; FY 1974 authorization was $30 million. The FY 1974 Congressional appropriation was $25 million. Significant amendments to the legislation have authorized provision of hospital services, inclusion of seasonal farm workers on a restricted basis, and has required consumer and community involvement in planning and implementing projects.

II. Program operations

In the last year of the undiluted "classical" MHP the average grant size was for $61,000, and 53 percent of grant funds went for projects worth less than $100,000. Fifty-seven percent of grant funds went to upstream projects, which are smaller on the average than home-base projects; home-base projects were of two basic sizes: one similar to the upstream projects, and another of about $200,000 size. Health departments sponsored 67 percent of the projects and received 75 percent of grant funds. There were no migrants found in the area; the larger projects covered no greater percentage of the migrant population in their area than the small ones. Thirty-seven different states received grants, twenty-five state health departments received grants for their consultation services for a total of $900,000, and including the funds they subgranted, the state health departments controlled $4.5 million, or over one-half of total program funds. The same pattern of operations can be discerned early in the program as well. Through the years the great majority of projects were retained in the program.

III. Project organization and operations

A. Project sampling reveals the following average figures for personnel: 14 percent of a project's funds are spent for physician outpatient services, almost invariably on a part-time basis. Two and one-half nurses are employed per project, and about twice as much is spent on nurses as doctors, for 25 percent of a project's budget. Two-thirds of all projects have at least one sanitarian, and 85 percent of health department sponsored projects have at least one. Only 28 percent of projects employed aides of any kind, and these were not generally recruited from the recipient population, and not used in an innovative way.

B. Project sampling reveals the following facts for medical care delivery: 80 percent of the projects offer general medical clinics, 52 percent offer fee-for-service referral, 20 percent exclusively the latter. Many offer health department type categorical clinics. Most home-base projects have daytime clinics, most upstream projects night clinics, often in makeshift offices in the camps. The clinics almost never have laboratory, X-ray, or EKG facilities on site. The physicians spend only a small amount of time with each patient. Nursing services are offered far in excess of physician services; nurses concentrate on case-finding, health education, and triage, to the exclusion of physician-initiated services.

C. Sanitarians practice the usual health department surveillance activities, to the exclusion of work with field sanitation, pesticide control, or occupational hazards. Neither laws nor the political environment vigorously support environmental improvement.

D. Both nurses and sanitarians indulge heavily in health education activities.

E. Over half the projects reviewed offer inpatient care services, and an average of 29 percent of the budget goes for this sector.

F. There was no evidence of the existence of formal or informal channels for consumer feedback.

IV. Program evaluation

In presentation to Congress, the MHP has traditionally cited two statistics: the number of services provided, and the number counties "covered." These statistics have questionable accuracy and have been used in a misleading fashion. There is no evidence of any serious internal evaluation effort, nor even collection of statistics, for the program or its projects. Applying the previously-derived causality scheme for migrant health shows that the "classical" MHP chose three causes for concentrated effort: mobility, environment, and medical care. It also concentrated on two "red herrings": health education and inter-project coordination. The program's approach to the three legitimate causes had very significant weaknesses: the environmental approach chose only to try weakly to enforce the existing laws; the medical care component supplied only poor-quality episodic, symptomatic physician care plus "health department" type preventive services; and the efforts made to combat the problems of mobility were vitiated by the poor quality, lack of comprehensiveness, and unacceptability of the medical services. The overall efficiency of operations was poor, since 19 percent of funds went for program level administration and state level consultations, medical care services were of poor quality, the environmental efforts were ill-founded, there was a poor component balance in projects (as with physician-nursing balances and inpatient-outpatient balances), there was little significant use of paramedical personnel, and the scale of operations was too small by about a factor of ten.

Chapter Three

Proposed Alternatives to the Classical Solution

This chapter presents and evaluates various alternatives to the "classical" Migrant Health Program (MHP). A great many possible combinations of approaches can be conjured up, but we shall limit our attention to only those strategies aimed specifically at the health of migrants—as opposed to such general programs as national health insurance, rural health programs, welfare reform, or job training—and only those programs that have been proposed at some time by persons concerned with the problem. The objectives are to gain perspective on these strategic possibilities vis-à-vis the root causes of ill health among migrants, and to find if any of the strategies is satisfactory for promoting with some confidence. These limitations are adopted because the basic purpose of the book is the practical one of taking a solid, incremental step forward in the MHP—and generating new alternatives at this point would be a chancy business, when the author knows from having done the analysis that there is indeed one that "satisfices."[a]

The alternatives we shall consider here are as follows:

1. Direct cash grant
2. Medical insurance
3. Referral activity
4. Hospitalization services only
5. Mothers and children
6. The stream approach—mobile clinics
7. Regional health centers

[a]This term, from *Administrative Behavior* by Herbert Simon, combines the words "satisfy" and "suffice." Simon contends that the search for alternatives in situations such as we have in this chapter, usually stops (and rightly so) when a solution "satisfices."

As explained in Chapter 2 (page 70) the programs will be ranked on a semi-quantitative scale by the author's judgment. Although readers will differ in rating the specific elements, it is hoped that the overall patterns evolved will achieve a rough consensus.

I DIRECT CASH GRANT

This approach is not strictly a "health program," but its simplicity and potential to be directed to health is so great that we do consider it here.

A. Rationale

Modern free enterprise economic ~~thought~~ theory says money is best spent directly by consumers, who can express their priorities as appropriate to them, without the waste of bureaucracy, the inevitably inappropriate choice of goods and services by administrators, and without paternalism and its deleterious side effects. What the government chooses to spend on health, a migrant himself might choose to spend on food, or clothing, or a TV set. What an administration spends on medical care, a migrant might spend on environmental improvement. The theory is that whatever he chooses, it's his life, and he should live it as best as he can choose. Decentralized decision-making is bound to be more efficient than centralized decision-making would be.

B. Causal Analysis

1. Poverty (++++). This factor, probably the most important of all in the production of poor health, is attacked head on by the direct grant approach. This is not to say poverty will be alleviated completely by this approach—that would depend on the amount of money involved. Nonetheless, insofar as money is granted at all, poverty is to some extent ameliorated. The probable direct connection between poverty and ill health is therefore favorably affected.

2. Mobility (0). This factor cannot be much affected by increased wealth. The incentive structure of the transfer payments (or other means of increasing the wealth of migrants) would determine whether they continued to migrate or not, but it would be unlikely that any method not involving direct alternative work training and placement provisions would halt the migratory patterns.

3. Discrimination (+). Discrimination seems to have an interactionary link with poverty. A decrease in poverty might well have some decrease in discrimination attendant upon it. We would expect, however, that such a decrease would be small, since socio-cultural-color-language problems would still remain in full force. Furthermore, the specific problem of discrimination in health resources—both environmental and medical care—would have no specific counterweighting force; that is to say, with the direct cash grant approach, no specific efforts would be made to counter the effects of discrimination in

decreasing the effective availability of medical care, and making the environment worse.

4. Rural Medical Care Capacity (0). This factor would remain unaffected by direct cash grants. The distribution of physicians has been relatively unresponsive to the potential money to be made in rural areas, and the increment of wealth migrants would add would be miniscule.

5. Environment (++). Increased wealth would be translated to some degree into improved environmental conditions. How much conditions would improve would depend a great deal on how much wealthier the migrants would become.

We listed on the causality scheme three causal conditions that lead to an unhealthy environment: poverty, discrimination and mobility. Direct cash grants affect mainly poverty, discrimination slightly, and mobility not at all. We would expect the environment to be improved in the elements for which poverty is the main precursor. The main improvements would come in the home-base housing units, over which the migrant himself has a great deal of control, and which are regarded as permanent abodes. Increased space per person, improvements in refrigeration, and improvements in human waste disposal would probably be the main elements affected. Relatively unaffected would be areas over which local governments have control, such as water supply, sewage disposal, etc. The main precursors for such deficiencies are probably discrimination and political impotence.

Field sanitation and upstream environmental conditions would also be unaffected. Field sanitation is under the control of the growers, who would have no reason to change. Upstream residences are more obviously temporary than home-base residences, and ownership is not lodged with the migrant. Increased wealth of the migrant might lead to rental of better homes on occasion, but the camps would almost certainly be unimproved. The owners of the camps are activated by many factors other than the wealth of the migrant in the condition in which they keep the camps. Some motivations we can identify would be, for instance, general prejudice and discrimination towards the migrant, long established custom, the accurate knowledge that even the small improvements sometimes made are often mistrated by the occupants (well explained by Coles), [1] intense competition for the grower's expenditure of any money by a multitude of areas that would benefit him directly, and lack of enforcement of laws (such as they are) on camp environment. On the migrant's side, there is little reason for him to invest time, money, and effort to improve an environment he will not be likely to see soon again. There is little reason to believe more money in the migrant's pocket, then, would improve his work camp conditions.

The improvement in environment resulting from increased wealth of the migrant would be, in sum, segmental, but important.

6. Occupational Hazards (0). There is no obvious way in which increased wealth of the migrant would be translated into decreased occupational

hazards, which are caused by inattention to safety standards by supervisory personnel and owners, and by lack of safety features on equipment supplied by manufacturers.

7. Malnutrition (++++). Increased wealth would have an immediate and pronounced effect on nutritional status. The Colorado Migrant Council study [2] cited earlier indicates a nutritionally rational choice of foods by migrants with increased money to spend, and increased wealth is usually associated with improved nutritional status. It is entirely likely that purchase of more and better quality food would be the first effect of increased wealth with this population.

8. Medical Care Provision (+). Although the availability of medical care in the areas of migrant permanent and temporary residence would not be improved, and the effects of mobility untempered, the migrants' increased wealth would enable them to purchase increased amounts when necessary. They probably would purchase a great deal;[3] the pattern of consumption would emphasize the episodic and emergent. Purchase of insurance would be unlikely. Hospitalization is so expensive that it would take an unreasonable increase in wealth for that avenue to be open to the migrant; to most Americans the hospital can only be countenanced with insurance protection. Health department services would be unchanged.

8a. Type of Medical Care Provided (0). The quality of care purchased would be likely to be rather worse than average. Discrimination would cause the migrant to be more than occasionally ill-served by physicians, probably, since the latter are well stocked with patients and can therefore call their patients by priority. Common experience tells us that medical ethics are a counterweight to such impulses, but hardly a pervasive one. Moreover, the quality of care even the middle class receives in rural areas is highly suspect, since the quality of physicians and hospitals there is not high, and the press of patients is intense. The comprehensiveness of services available would be limited by the providers, and thus be low. Accessibility would be a severe problem. The episodic and emergent pattern is neither desirable nor efficient.

The fact that the migrants would be served by the same system of care serving everyone else would have a variable effect on dignity and acceptability. Whereas some would experience degrading discrimination, others would be able to feel the satisfaction of equal treatment and equal care.

9. Efficiency (+++). Administrative efficiency is one of the most attractive aspects of the cash grant scheme. Although, like any scheme, it could be made top heavy in practice by many rules, much paper, a means test, large number of disbursements per year, etc., it could as well be very simple, concerning itself only with identifying the recipients and giving them their money once or twice a year.

To the extent that the money would later be spent on medical care, an element of inefficiency might be introduced. As has been explained above, the medical care received might well be of inferior quality as well as rather high priced. On the other hand, few programs could be so efficient in improving nutrition, allowing for individual tastes.

10. Spillover (++). Since the recipients of the grants would be free to use the money however they wanted, there would surely be many effects on their lives from areas other than health. Some of these other effects would not be spillover effects, strictly speaking, since they would not be incurred along with, but rather instead of better health. A true spillover effect would be self-esteem that would not be lost, and self-reliance not undercut by undue interference by government officials.

C. Discussion

The cash grant approach chooses probably the most important precursor to poor health and hits it hard. Several intermediary steps are affected in the process. There seems to be, however, an entire area of action that is very little affected—that of medical care. If medical care were of very little importance for good health, the cash grant approach would be quite appropriate; if medical care were of great importance for good health, the cash grant approach would be quite inappropriate. To which end of the spectrum the true situation lies we do not know, but most people would say medical care is important. Furthermore, "effective" or not, medical care is apparently a much desired item, therefore it must be "useful" in some sense, and a case would be made for a positive role of social policy in supplying it. The cash grants approach would not supply medical care well.

Another way of looking at this approach is as follows: to be effective, a program must devote its resources to the "bottlenecks" that is, the most important identified causes of ill health, the ones that are "limiting" at the moment. The whole idea of cash grants is the micro-economic insight that a family almost tautologically spends money in the marginally most efficient place. This analysis assumes the social-economic system and institutions remain as they are, and that all necessary goods and services are purchasable, or potentially purchasable if demand develops sufficiently. If the "bottleneck" is really the system, however, which is somehow refractory to the economic demand in question, then the above reasoning does not work out so well.

(A further consideration is that although the theory says that the system will change in accordance with dollar incentives, the migrants could not be counted upon to be powerful bidders even with more dollars, and in medical care the system has not played a micro-economic role well at all. Theory further states that if migrants cannot bid well for medical care, then it is more important for society to serve the more powerful bidders anyway, since they are more productive. We would reject this theoretical view for a more equalitarian and humanitarian one.)

If the "bottleneck" is medical care, then it is a system change that is needed, and the rural health care system, along with the overall health care system, has proved pretty clearly to be not controllable through the market mechanism. Similarly, the area of environment is not simply a case of the market. To pass new laws, enforce old ones, and supply governmental services, collective action would seem to be insufficient.

On the other hand, it is quite possible that we have underestimated the power of the direct cash approach. There are so many imponderables it is hard to tell. Usually a rise in economic status is associated with improved environmental conditions (perhaps caused by pathways not yet defined–decreased family size, decreased discrimination, increased educational status, and increased political power. The question of "chicken and egg" causal connections is undefined here).

Would all of the above accrue from direct cash transfers? We have no examples of such a thing happening. The American value system would be unlikely to grant social rewards to those who were the fortunate objects of "charity." The funds might be resented by the recipients. It might be possible to disguise the transfer by subsidizing wages and creating jobs for the unemployed, thus making the gains non-charitable. There is just a lot here we don't know; this approach could be a lot better than we think.

In any event, the amount of money involved would be crucial. The current migrant health appropriation would supply about $100 per family, with non-migrant seasonal farm workers completely excluded. Taking the OEO Title III-B and ESEA Title I program appropriations together with Migrant Health (assuming they would adopt the same reasoning) brings us to about $400–$500 per family. While an improvement of $500 per year income would be significant, representing about a 17 percent improvement of the average, probably, a quadrupling of this amount of money would raise the average yearly income to $5,000. With such sums available, few would want to channel the migrant's expenditures for him; why, he would be middle class! Having reached the limits of health considerations, we must stop speculation at this point.

Causal Profile Summary:

(1)	(2)	(3)	(4)	(5)	(6)	(7)	(8)	(8a)	(9)	(10)
++++	0	+	0	++	0	++++	+	0	+++	++

II MEDICAL INSURANCE

The Office of Economic Opportunity contracted with Control Systems Research, Inc., for a migrant health insurance feasibility study, which was presented in 1971.[4] This sensitive study posited a program with the following characteristics: operating on an interstate basis; administered independently of farm employers; not contingent on employment status; covering work-related accidents and injuries; ensuring free choice of provider; involving a simple, immediate, and direct claims procedure; and requiring voluntary participation. Such a program did appear feasible to the contractors, and they asserted that a demonstration should be conducted. Unfortunately, one never was, but this study offers a useful prototype for our theoretical analysis.

A. Rationale

The insurance approach rests on the belief that medical care is very important for migrants' health, and that medical insurance provides the best access for the migrant to the medical care dispensing system.

> The migrant population is decreasing. In the last 20 years, the total farm labor force has been decreasing; the migratory worker population has been decreasing at a similar rate. . . .
>
> The migrant population is dispersed. Although migrants concentrate in crop areas where hand harvesting or cultivating is required, within these areas they are dispersed through many counties. In only 40 of the nation's 3100 counties do migrants concentrate in numbers of 5000 or more.
>
> Migrants are mobile. In following the season, they range from the southern parts of California, Texas and Florida to Washington, Michigan and New York. . . . The health needs of the migrant population cannot be scheduled to coincide with the locations of migrant health programs.
>
> Given the nature of migrant life, and the inherent difficulties in providing direct service programs for a shrinking, mobile and dispersed population, health insurance may offer a more flexible mechanism for financing the delivery of health care to the *entire* migrant population. It recognizes a simple fact of life: in most areas of the migrant streams, the only source of health care is the private health care system or the public hospital. Whether health insurance would in fact be useful to the migrant population is something which has yet to be demonstrated.[5]

The type of insurance plan propounded, however, would have to differ considerably from a commercial-type plan.

> (The) concern is to promote access to health services, not to protect against catastrophic loss. . . . (In commercial policies) restrictions have been placed to protect the underwriter against 'adverse cost experience'; we are interested in having the migrants protect themselves against 'adverse health experience'.[6]

B. Causal Analysis

1. Poverty (0). Except in the sense that under this program some services would be paid for, thus furnishing in-kind income, this program would have no effect on the problem of poverty among migrants.

2. Mobility (+). The insurance program adapts to the migrants' mobility by making payment for care applicable no matter where the migrant might be at any time. Great barriers deriving from the mobile condition would still remain, however; any insurance program would have to decide whether to try to help the migrants overcome these residual barriers. The proposed OEO program decided not to:

> Our approach in overcoming the non-financial barriers to health care is to provide an opportunity for the migrants to learn through their own experiences with health care providers. We have rejected the missionary approach of telling or "educating" migrants about what constitutes good health and when they should visit the doctor. Migrants have been victims of this particularly annoying form of condescending benevolence in so many other areas of their life that they would tune out faster than they could be "referred to an appropriate medical resource." Migrants should have the opportunity to encounter the private health care system as it is, and thereby learn what they must do for themselves.[7]

3. Discrimination (0). There is nothing in this program that would alleviate discrimination on any but a financial basis, although it is true that by providing the migrants with a basis for payment that is similar to that used by middle-class people, one is possibly helping them to be regarded as the same as other people.

4. Medical Care Capacity (0). One of the prime criticisms of the insurance approach is that it can have no positive effect on the underlying problem of insufficient medical care capacity. (We have described previously how demand increase does not seem to stimulate supply increase in medical care, especially in rural areas.) Care that is delivered to migrants will therefore be to some extent robbed from Peter to pay Paul, and will also suffer from high prices and low quality as well, in all likelihood.

The OEO study confronted this problem directly. First, they considered the relationship of insurance to migrant health clinics. They concluded that "the . . . likely pattern would be for migrants to use migrant health clinics where they are available and private health facilities in other areas."[8] Eventually, they came to consider that a good

> . . . strategy would involve a reorientation of the direct service programs. The bulk of the direct service program funds could be channeled into home base clinics whose job it would be to service the migrants who concentrate in the home base area for five to seven months. The clinics would enroll migrants in the health insurance program, which migrants could use upstream in the working areas or enroute thereto. (The insurance could be usable downstream as

well.) Certain upstream direct service programs in areas of favorable private provider distribution could be phased out.[9]

Largely because of the shortage of medical resources in home-base areas, then, the OIO study suggested that insurance be used only in conjunction with what we refer to as regional health centers.

5. Environment (0). This insurance approach can have no effect on environmental problems.

6. Occupational Hazard Alleviation (0). No effect.

7. Malnutrition (0). No effect.

8. Medical Care Provision (++++). This factor is of course at the heart of the insurance approach. To the extent that money can buy medical care in the areas where migrants find themselves, they would be able to afford themselves of care. Criterion number 4, of course, speaks to the fact that in many areas care is unpurchasable, and the insurance approach would be of little avail in such areas.

8a. Type of Medical Care Provided (0). The specific services offered could vary widely under this program. Typically, however, insurance programs stress therapeutic efforts over regular preventive care, and make no effort to structure a system of access to care for the patient. Also typically, insurance benefits have regulations that induce inefficiencies—hospitalization is favored over outpatient treatment, for instance. Insurance programs also typically favor more rather than less treatment—probably a salubrious effect for the chronically undertreated migrants. The other side of that balance, however, would be struck by deductible and co-insurance provisions that virtually every insurance policy has. An OEO type program would minimize the disadvantageous attributes, but many would remain.

The technical quality of care the migrant received would be dependent upon the physicians into whose office he happened. As has been mentioned several times, that quality would in most instances be low, although not so low as in the clinics held by the classical program. The amenities of service would likely be particularly better, although discrimination would be a stumbling block. Comprehensiveness and accessibility would be likely to be low.

In general, the insurance approach would deliver to the migrant the same kind of care delivered to rural populations, subject to alteration by the other causal factors not approached by the program. Whether such care is good enough or not must be a major policy decision.

9. Efficiency (0). Fee-for-service payments at a distance with many rules—the financing mechanism utilized by medical insurance that does not relate to a prepayment plan—has been a system frequently criticized for theoretical and practical inefficiency, although of course there must be a range of efficiency according to the specifics of the various plans. On the other hand, the insurance scheme would enable migrants to insert themselves in ongoing eco-

nomies of scale that might exist. Prices indicate, howerver, that such economies should they exist are not passed on to the consumer in any case, with the possible exception of some of the prepaid plans. The paperwork inefficiency component would no doubt be substantial, and inefficiencies in patient convenience would be substantial, especially since long rides to find providers would be expected.

10. Spillover Effects (0). The insurance approach would have very few spillover effects. It is difficult to envision how new jobs in any substantial numbers could be created for migrants, or how any community organization or economic progress could be effected.

C. Discussion

The basic approach of the insurance scheme, then, is limited almost entirely to the provision of medical care. The method of provision would by direct purchase on a fee-for-service basis from the current system as it exists. Discounted is the contribution to ill health of the numerous other factors we have mentioned. Discounted also are the tremendous problems associated with purchase of care from the current system: frequently poor quality, high prices, no emphasis on prevention, unavailability, etc. Discounted also are the inefficiencies attendant on payment from third party sources on a fee-for-service basis. It would seem most unlikely that health insurance alone would do a great deal to improve the migrants' state of health. It is possible, however, that such an approach might be fruitful as an adjunct to a basically different program, and might cover migrants in areas rather well supplied medically.

Causal Profile Summary:

(1)	(2)	(3)	(4)	(5)	(6)	(7)	(8)	(8a)	(9)	(10)
0	+	0	0	0	0	0	++++	0	0	0

III REFERRAL ACTIVITY

Referral activity would consist of identifying the migrant and his problem, and sending him to the proper public or private agency(ies) or practitioner(s) for solution of that problem. Payment for the services dispensed could also be partially or wholly paid for by the program, in several different ways. A variant of the scheme, actually put into practice on the East Coast by a grant in FY 1970, would identify resources by region as well as by local area and try to move the resource and the person together.

A. Rationale

The traditional rationale for referral agencies is that resources to help people exist, but they are hard to locate and it is difficult to cut through the red tape. A central clearinghouse can act as a catalyst to bring together resource and needy person. Paying for the service in behalf of the person is an addition to the basic concept of catalyst, and amends the basic concept somewhat, admitting that resources as provided by the public sector are sometimes deficient, but asserting instead that where such deficiencies exist the "gap can be plugged" by purchase of private services.

Historically, the referral approach to medical care for migrants was the keystone of the Agricultural Workers Health and Medical Association of the Farm Security Administration in the late 1930s and 1940s. Milton I. Roemer, now Professor of Public Health at UCLA, and formerly an employee of the Farm Security Administration, speaks well of AWHMA, extolling particularly the economies of having a nurse do preliminary triage.[10] On the other hand, it is clear that AWHMA could not and did not aim to provide comprehensive care to the patients, but mostly episodic medical care as demanded (see Chapter 1, pp. 14–15).

Referral is a not inconsequential part of the "classical" program's activities.

B. Causal Analysis

1. Poverty (0). No direct attempt is made to intervene in the economic status of the migrants.

2. Mobility (++). Referral activities make allowance for the migrants' mobile status. Good outreach efforts could feed right into referral activities, both locally and regionally.

3. Discrimination (0). Special efforts would be made to seek out migrants and place them with a selected service dispenser. On the other hand, placement in public agencies for service is itself discriminatory since such agencies were set up and are run separately and unequally.

4. Rural Medical Care Capacity (0). Referral activities would have no positive effect on developing increased capacity of the medical care system.

5. Environment (0). There would be no effect on the environment by referral activities.

6. Occupational Hazards (0). There would be no effect on occupational hazards by referral activities.

7. Malnutrition Alleviation (0). There might be an effect on malnutrition if that were a recognized problem with a case, and there were resources available to ameliorate the problem. The availability of such resources would be problematical.

8. Medical Care Provision (++++). Provision of medical care is at the heart of the referral approach. The major problem would be that criterion 4 speaks to the problem of the lack of purchasability of medical care in a great many of the areas. Furthermore, as has been pointed out earlier, such public resources for medical care provision that do exist often find migrants ineligible for service.

8a. Type of Medical Care Provided (0). The referral approach must be primarily geared to providing episodic, acute care plus certain basic categorical services such as well-baby examinations. Such categorical services would be only lightly used, since the great expenditure of time, energy, and money to complete many such visits would be prohibitive. The quality of the services delivered would be variable, although as with the insurance approach a high level would not be expected. With limited funds some manner of rationing of services would inevitably appear; the rationing method decided on would probably affect quality adversely. The type of service provided, then, would be primarily acute care, with the providers being first such public agencies as exist (categorical clinics certain to be poorly utilized), and then the same private practitioners who service the rest of the population. The services offered and the number of visits allowed would be limited. The referral makers would be in a position to decide on a case-by-case basis what was rational and what was not, as well as to choose specific physicians. The impact of this latter would be, however, questionable. Accessibility would be fairly good, but acceptability, with many stops before receiving care, and utilizing many degrading services for the poor, would not.

9. Efficiency (+). Two obvious sources of efficiency would be avoidance of service delivery by overqualified personnel, since patients would be screened, and utilization of low-cost services where available. On the other hand, patients would often be inconvenienced by multiple stops before completion of treatment, prices encoutered in the private market place would be high, and the services received would not be preventive. Furthermore, there are in fact but few public low-cost resources to be used, even if one looks for them.

10. Spillover Effects (0). Only few spillover effects would be noted from the referral program, and these would not be necessary, but optional. Aides could be enlisted for outreach, creating new jobs and skills, but only a few. Some of them would obtain a working knowledge of the operation of county services that would lead to an increased sophistication in the migrant community about social and governmental workings. But these gains would be optional, and small.

C. Discussion

The worst problem with referral approach is that it is based in the first instance on a delusion that appropriate and acceptable social and medical services for migrants exist, if only these services could be found and obtained. There simply are very, very few such services. Referrals would usually come to the local practitioners. The referral system, if conducted by competent medical personnel, could treat some of the patients without recourse to physicians, and could make referrals to the proper specialist appropriately. The services would be costly, of questionable quality, and difficult to obtain in many areas. Certainly no progressive solution to the problem of declining rural medical service capacity would be offered. Rather, the same old system would be further taxed. Furthermore, as with the insurance approach, little note would be taken of the many other important causes of poor health besides lack of medical care. In sum, the referral approach would have something to offer in areas of abundant medical care, if quality and price could be controlled. But the problems associated with the approach make it an unlikely choice for a main theme of approach to migrant health.

Causal Profile Summary:

(1)	(2)	(3)	(4)	(5)	(6)	(7)	(8)	(8a)	(9)	(10)
0	++	0	0	0	0	+	++++	0	+	0

IV HOSPITALIZATION SERVICES ONLY

This approach would envision a patient reporting to a local triage center when ill, probably at the local hospital. There the patient would be evaluated possibly by a physician or retainer, to determine whether or not he needed admission to the hospital. If the patient fell into a category defined by the program as reimbursable, he would be admitted and treated. Services would be rendered for surgical and medical emergencies, for serious illnesses, and possibly for childbirths, and elective surgery.

A. Rationale

The rationale for this approach rests on the assumption that the most important and effective treatments for the most important diseases are rendered in hospitals, that most diseases seen in primary care are self-limited and thus need not be seen and treated and most serious diseases are not preventable even if early symptoms are detected, so all resources should be concentrated on the highly productive hospital sector.

B. Causal Analysis

1. Poverty (0). No direct effect.

2. Mobility (0). A positive effect only in the sense that the migrant would be able to avail himself of hospital care wherever he would go, but this is minimal.

3. Discrimination (0). A positive effect only in the sense that any program that is specifically for migrants to some extent counters the effect of discrimination.

4. Rural Medical Care Capacity (0). No effect.

5. Environment (0). No effect.

6. Occupational Hazard Alleviation (0). No effect.

7. Malnutrition (0). No effect.

8. Medical Care Provision (++++). The entire thrust of this approach is on the direct provision of medical care. Little difficulty would be encountered in providing the services, since medical care facilities are in relatively abundant

supply in rural areas, and physicians are generally eager to care for remunerative and "interesting" hospital cases.

8a. Type of Medical Care Provided (+). Only a small segment of the usual spectrum of medical care services would be provided. The whole idea is that by *not* being comprehensive in the scope of services, the dross of medical care can be eliminated, and only effective procedures included. The quality of hospital services would generally be higher than we would expect in an office visit because of the informal and formal controls found in the hospital setting (e.g., visibility, peer pressure, tissue committees), even if rural hospitals are often small and inferior in quality as compared to most hospitals, and rural practitioners are thought to be inferior to those in non-rural areas. Identifying and locating hospitals and finding transportation to them might complicate accessibility, but at least hospitals are visible institutions and easier to locate than private offices.

The acceptability of services would be variable. Large institutions, especially those that have a long record of mistreating migrants, would be intimidating, and services rendered there might well be demeaning. Certainly, the language problems would be difficult to solve, and no representatives of the migrant population would be expected to be employed by this plan. If the past is any guide, acceptability would not be high.

9. Efficiency (0). Inefficiencies would accrue from the inevitable "fudging" of criteria and diagnoses, and treating patients as inpatients who could be dealt with more efficiently as outpatients. In addition, passing papers back and forth to certify and reimburse for each case would be inefficient. Finally, to the extent that the assumptions of this approach are wrong, and early diagnosis leads to more efficient care than late diagnosis, and treatments outside of the hospital are in fact more efficient than those inside the hospital, the plan is inherently inefficient. On the other hand, the quality of care would be better than for many plans emphasizing outpatient care in physicians offices.

10. Spillover Effects (0). There would be very few opportunities to introduce positive side effects into this program.

C. Discussion

The hospitalization argument says that the most cost-effective services in medical care are rendered in the hospital. Therefore, since funds are quite limited, they should be concentrated in supporting hospital care. But are hospital services the most cost-effective? Conventional wisdom states otherwise. Some diseases can be prevented altogether, others can be best treated in early stages. Some diseases might not be so serious in their ultimate threat to life and function, but they are relatively well and cheaply controlled, whereas many more serious diseases requiring hospitalization are expensive to treat, but are nearly hopeless therapeutically. Finally, hospitals treat some rather unserious diseases, such as hernias, whereas many serious disorders, such as diabetes and hypertension, are treated outside the hospital. For the hospitalization argument to be proved correct, careful studies would have to be done for these conventional arguments, especially convincing with the young age group represented by migrant workers and their families, to be upset. Were a list of priorities for cost-effective practices in medicine to be developed, it would be unlikely that hospital treatments would be found predominantly at the top.

Practically, there would certainly be a great deal of "fudging"; physicians will do whatever is necessary to treat (and receive reimbursement for) a patient that medical science says should be treated. Indeed, the physician's training as a professional emphasizes that his responsibility is to the patient, no matter what bureaucratic rules are promulgated. Under this hospitalization plan, many patients who could be treated as outpatients would instead be cared for in a much more expensive way.

Many of the emergency cases that this program would cover would probably have been cared for anyway, since many hospitals recognize their public responsibility to serve those needing care without regard to reimbursement possibilities. On the other hand, it is common practice in many areas to turn away such cases, and banking on free hospital treatment is demeaning, increases discrimination and prejudicial feelings, and decreases the quality of care.

Another consideration is the number of persons who could be served. If the average hospitalization were to cost $1,000, not a high figure, particularly if one includes the indirect costs in this scheme, only 25,000 patients could have been cared for in fiscal year 1974, for example or 2.5 percent of an estimated one million total migrant population. If one includes seasonal farm workers the figure drops to below 1 percent. Both these figures are fewer in number than the number of babies that would be born. An upper limit on allowable expenditures per patient could be made, but concentrating on expensive hospital care inevitably means delivering care to only a few persons.

Most of the arguments presented above persuade the author that hospitalization only would be a difficult plan to carry out, and that it offers insufficient theoretical appeal to attempt. If one is to deliver medical care, it seems more appropriate to offer a comprehensive range of services, so long as one type of service does not seem to be particularly more cost-effective than any other. There still seems to be, moreover, no rationale to neglect the non-medical care precursors to bad health.

Causal Profile Summary:

(1)	(2)	(3)	(4)	(5)	(6)	(7)	(8)	(8a)	(9)	(10)
0	0	0	0	0	0	0	++++	+	0	0

V MOTHERS AND CHILDREN

By this plan persons eligible for services would be limited only to children and mothers, although services to that group would be comprehensive. Provision of services could be either by clinic or referral, but most proposers of this plan have clinics in mind, and the discussion here shall be of clinics.

A. Rationale

Given that funds are less than adequate to cover the whole migrant population, it is best to limit one's aims. Rather than decrease the number of services offered across the board, it is better to single out a group of importance to receive the full range of services, since delivering less than the full range decreases efficiency. Women and children are selected since a healthy mother is necessary for rearing healthy children, and it is supposed that giving preventive and therapeutic care, in addition to health education to children, will lead to less care being necessary for them as adults. It is also thought desirable that care of children pays off for a longer time, for children will live longer than their parents (discounting for the lag before economic productivity begins is neglected in this argument.)

B. Causal Analysis

1. Poverty (0). No effect.

2. Mobility (++). Positive effects by setting up specific sites of care for the migrants, and outreach (as with "classical" program).

3. Discrimination (0). No effect, except insofar as services are provided selectively for this population.

4. Rural Medical Care Capacity (?). There might be some positive effect on the rural medical care capacity. It might be possible to lure outside physicians to rural areas to work in maternal and child projects, but probably only in special cases where a national recruitment effort were to be mounted. It would also be possible, depending on the nature of the centers, that changes in organization would be made that would improve productivity. Use of nonprofessional personnel and a form of group practice would also be possible.

It is important, however, to distinguish between what would be possible and what would be necessarily implied in a program. It would be *possible* to incorporate these features in a maternal and child care center, but it would be just as *possible* to run clinics with local physicians hurrying through as many patients as possible once a week, as the "classical" program did. Therefore, since the population limitation proposal is only really a fragmentary proposal, we must acknowledge that the "rural medical care capacity" factor would have wide variability, and thus cannot be rated.

5. Environmental Improvement (0). No effect.

6. Occupational Hazards (0). No effect.

7. Malnutrition (+). There might be some effect on this factor, since nutrition is a primary factor that a maternal and child clinic would want to concentrate on. Since poverty is the main precursor of malnutrition, however, it would be unlikely for clinics to make much of an impact, unless there were large provisions for food supplements. A clinic that interpreted its responsibilities broadly might make a significant impact by involving local food stamp offices, but history shows that instances of such bureaucratic cooperation are rare.

8. Medical Care (++++). Dispensing medical care is the major focus of this approach. The organized approach to the provision of medical care releases the migrants from the necessity of seeking care from the already overburdened system themselves; the possibility of increased productivity by physician recruitment and progressive organization would enhance the chances of large amounts of medical care being delivered.

8a. Type of Medical Care Provided (?). Comprehensive services would be delivered to the non-comprehensive population covered. The quality, accessibility, and acceptability of the services would be dependent on many factors, according to the specifics of the program.

9. Efficiency (?). There would be potential for this program to be quite efficient; most of the money could go directly to services without diversion to billing procedures and forms. However, depending on the organization of the services and their quality, efficiency could be poor. Once again, this program cannot be rated because of the fragmentary nature of the proposal.

10. Spillover Effects (?). There would be ample opportunity to build in numerous spillover effects to a maternal and child care approach. Non-professional personnel could be recruited from the consumer populations, thus providing jobs and alternative careers for them. In addition, a well-organized and aggressive center could well act as advocate for its patients in the community in a number of ways. On the other hand, none of this could apply.

C. Discussion

This program has never been proposed in more than the outline form presented here. Like the hospitalization only proposal, it seeks to limit those receiving benefits in a rational manner. It reasons that one cannot select a certain sector of the population-at-risk that should receive priority. In fact, however, this proposal is less drastic than it sounds, since by one estimate about 70 percent of the migrant population is composed of mothers and children,[11] since it is always relatively easier to get mothers and children to go to clinics than adult males, and since the need for care generally centers around that population anyway. Viewed from that aspect, much of the logic of the population restriction vanishes. For if an adult male comes to a clinic with a complaint, the odds say that one should pay attention to him, for he does not do so lightly. By making such a person ineligible for services, one would not only be missing important illnesses, but by officially sanctioning exclusion of men, one would also be making more difficult patient attraction when full services for all were introduced.

A further hole in the logic favoring the treatment of children comes from ignoring the discount factor. Although treating a child now will leave him with his whole working life ahead to produce without handicap, he must wait until he is a proper age to work. A currently working man can produce right away. This time difference makes it not nearly so obvious as it sometimes seems that a child is more important than a man. Even if the two assumptions made by this proposal are correct—that marginal utility increases as more services are given to a population, and that mothers and children are the most important group to be served—nevertheless, these other considerations make it clear that formally limiting services to just mothers and children would be a mistake.

Causal Profile Summary:

(1)	(2)	(3)	(4)	(5)	(6)	(7)	(8)	(8a)	(9)	(10)
0	++	0	?	0	0	+	++++	?	?	?

VI THE STREAM APPROACH—MOBILE CLINICS

Medical care under the system of mobile clinics would be dispensed from trailers containing medical equipment and examining rooms and staffed by a permanent team of medical personnel. The entire clinic would locate itself in the home-base areas during the winter and would follow the stream of migrants north during the warmer months. The trailers would contain laboratory, X-ray, and electrocardiograph equipment. The teams could be variously composed, but would include at least doctors and nurses, and probably laboratory technicians. The mobile clinics would refer patients to local specialists where indicated.

A. Rationale

Mobile clinics are often the first solution to the migrant health problem that comes to mind. Mobility is the most obvious distinguishing characteristic of the migrants when one considers them abstractly (when confronted in person, the racial, ethnic, and economic characteristics are more obvious than mobility), and mobile clinics would seem to cater directly to that point of uniqueness. The problem of overwhelmed local medical systems would be obviated by having the migrants bring along their own medical personnel and facilities, and both equipment and personnel of the MHP could be used full time no matter what the season. Furthermore, continuity of care would improve, since clinics would try to follow a group continuously.

B. Causal Analysis

1. Poverty (0). No direct effect.

2. Mobility (0). It is the factor of mobility that stimulates the idea of this program. Migrants however, do not travel in stable and discrete streams, but rather in very individualistic patterns that are often spontaneously impro-

vised. Although it can be predicted with some certainty how many migrants will come to a certain area, it cannot be predicted which individuals these migrants will be. It would be impossible, then, for a mobile unit to deliver continuous care to a group of migrants.

Neither would accessibility of health services be aided by mobile units traveling up and down the streams. In each new location the unit would have to find the migrants, establish and publicize a schedule for efficient visiting, and find appropriate locations for proper water and electricity hookups. These jobs are difficult enough to do for permanent residents; a short-time visitor in an area would be lucky just to find one suitable spot for the whole stay. And if it did find a permanent spot, it would then have to arrange outreach and transportation for its patients. In terms of access, this approach would be clearly inferior to even the "classical" program.

Mobile clinics might conceivably be more useful when used in concert with a local stationary system. Even in that instance, however, a significant improvement in accessibility would be doubtful. In East Africa, where extensive use has been made of mobile units in the context of a permanently situated main regional center, mobile units are used because the primitive transportation systems enforce an isolation upon widely dispersed rural residents far more severe than anything known to the United States.[12] The choice in Uganda and Kenya for rural residents has been between something and nothing. Travel conditions and population density in the United States are such that permanent centers within relatively easy reach of virtually all area residents can be established and permanent centers are to be preferred where they are possible.[13]

3. Discrimination (0). This program cannot be said to offer any antidote to discrimination. It is true that special services are provided just for the migrants, thus ensuring that they will not be excluded. Mobile clinics, however, have a distinct aura of second class medicine. A separate but unequal system cannot be said to be improving problems with discrimination. On the other hand, the personnel would be working only with migrants, and would be presumably sympathetic.

4. Rural Medical Care Capacity (+). For the times of clinic operation new personnel would be introduced in the area, if the personnel were to come along with the clinic as we have been supposing, the medical care capacity of the area would be improved. There would be no new organization to improve capacity, and the permanent impact on capacity would be null. In the case where the clinics were to be manned by local personnel, moreover, the impact would be null all year around.

5. Environment (0). No effect. Even if one were to try to build in an environmental component, the likelihood of success would be low, since sustained local efforts are necessary, rather than sporadic clean-up campaigns or such, here and there.

6. Occupational Hazards (0). No effect.

7. Malnutrition (0). No effect.

8. Medical Care Provision (++++). This program relies primarily on direct provision of medical care to improve the health status of the migrants. By providing that care directly, rather than merely providing the financial resources necessary to purchase care, the program insures that such care is in fact delivered.

8a. Type of Medical Care Provided (0). The program aims to deliver general acute medical care, although some preventive medicine could also be included. Although at first glance it would seem the program would provide good continuity of care, arguments made under point 2 above indicate that in fact continuity would be quite low. Although specialist referrals would of course be possible, the general thrust of the program would inexorably be toward only acute, and not in depth, care.

The quality of care delivered would be relatively low for several reasons. Not only would the care be focused on the acute, to the neglect of chronic conditions, in-depth diagnosis and treatment, and the preventive approach, but moreover, time and location problems would make access to care for acute conditions problematical. The great majority of spells of illness would be treated perforce in one or two visits, which would entail low quality for a significant number of illnesses. The organizational setting of one or two physicians divorced from any professional overview or specialist support would also tend to encourage low quality.

The amenities of service would also be lacking. Trailers have little space for awaiting and such services preclude the possibility of appointments. Long waiting times under the trees would hardly be considered adequate conditions. On the other hand, acceptability of services would be enhanced by the probable positive staff attitudes, and by the lack of intimidating appearances.

The comprehensiveness of services would undoubtedly be severely restricted by the scale of operations, the general intent of the program to simply provide a sick-call clinic, and the isolation of this component of service from others. "Mobile units (are) most applicable to periodic health services employing simple facilities, but (are) not desirable for Comprehensive Care."[14]

In sum, neither quality, nor comprehensiveness, nor accessibility would be very good at all; acceptability would be fair.

9. Efficiency (0). One rationale for the mobile stream approach was efficiency. Equipment could be used full time, instead of laying idle when the migrants were away. Personnel, likewise, could be employed full time. These gains, however, would be counterbalanced by other losses. Upkeep, coordination, and depreciation costs would be high. The small units of operation would bring inefficiency. Most importantly, the type of care delivered would be so low in quality, comprehensiveness, and accessibility that whatever the cost, efficiency would have to be rated low.

10. Spillover Effects (0). There would be a possibility for some

small spillover effects, but they would be quite limited in nature. Employment of migrants in nonprofessional capacities in mobile teams could be accomplished, but little education and upgrading could be done in these groups.

C. Discussion

One must question the assumption made by this approach that delivering medical care is the best way to improve the health of migrant workers. One must also question the assumption that the factor of mobility is the crucial problem in delivering health care to migrants. And even if those two assumptions were correct, the means used to combat mobility would be ineffective, as the above analysis shows. Only the idea of equipment and personnel transfer with the seasonal changes—by some other means than mobile units—seems to have potential usefulness.

Although somewhat different questions arise in considering using mobile clinics in a single local area, Bodenheimer (see note 12) clearly indicates that such arrangements are generally inefficient and ineffective. Only developing countries with their dearth of resources utilize mobile clinics, and even there, transition to permanent installations is counted as a major step forward.

Causal Profile Summary:

(1)	(2)	(3)	(4)	(5)	(6)	(7)	(8)	(8a)	(9)	(10)
0	+	0	+	0	0	0	++++	0	0	0

VII REGIONAL HEALTH CENTERS

This proposal contemplates building large centers for dispensing primary medical care, ancillary medical services, and environmental services in selected areas of major migrant impact. The medical organization would be based on the group practice principle with several physicians and many nurses and paraprofessionals. Outreach efforts and possible patient transportation systems would complement the medical effort. Environmental and occupational conditions would be part of the Center's concern. Exactly what action would be taken would vary according to the determination of each center individually.

Project location would be largely home base, where migrants are found for the longest periods of time and in the highest concentrations. Upstream, and mixed areas would also be eligible for such centers, according to the number of persons involved and the concentration of non-migrant seasonal farm workers. These major centers would be operated year around, with variations of capacity adjusted in concordance with impact seasons.

The regional health center proposal must also deal with the areas that could not be covered by a major center. Several alternatives would be available. If the area in question were located near enough to a major center, temporary or permanent satellites offering basic services could be set up using the major center as base and backup. In areas too far from major centers to coordinate closely, acute care centers could be set up to operate several times a week during peak load times, but relying on the major centers for the more comprehensive services, especially prevention. These temporary centers could also serve as follow-up centers for patients with chronic diseases treated at major centers at their home-base area. A third possibility for the lower impact areas would be building of year-round comprehensive services for migrants by providing services for a great many local residents by joint funding of projects, or just by buying into ongoing group practices, medical care foundations, or Health Maintenance organizations. A fourth possibility would be coverage by health insurance as detailed in Chapter 3, part III.

Many possible record and information systems have been suggested: patient-carried records; computer-stored records at a central facility with a toll-free telephone number; and record retention by the home-base facility, which would be responsible for coordinating all care for its patients. The last scheme is most feasible in the short run.

In 1970 about seven (depending on definition) centers resembling those suggested here were funded in home-base, upstream, and mixed areas in a marked departure from "classical" policies. The centers were each conceived as isolated projects rather than all being considered as components in an integrated system, none had a significant environmental component, and other aspects of the regional health center approach were not implemented. Unfortunately, these centers have not yet been subject to evaluation.

A. Rationale

This proposal rests on the conviction that comprehensive and in-depth health services, besides being cost-efficient, are necessary for services to have important and lasting results. It opts for giving fewer persons more and better services rather than giving more persons less and worse care. A few large centers are chosen rather than many smaller ones because of the economies of scale inherent in the larger operations. The existing medical care system is regarded as insufficient in capacity and quality to accommodate the migrants, and is thus avoided in both center and non-center areas. The proposal asserts the interdependence of medical care and environmental conditions, and contends it is synergistic to provide both these services together. The various schemes for non-center areas are proposed because of the necessity to treat acute disease wherever it occurs, and to provide for follow-up of chronic conditions treated primarily in the large centers.

B. Causal Analysis

1. Poverty (0). This approach entails no direct steps to improve poverty.

2. Mobility (++). This program adapts to migrants mobility in several ways. Conceding the difficulties of reaching and treating them while on the move, it seeks to maximize impact while they are stationary, hoping that as a result fewer problems will arise during transience, and that treatment of chronic conditions on the road will be mostly follow-ups. The various alternatives for the lower impact areas would seek to ameliorate transiency by outreach and, in the case of insurance, widespread applicability. Making the home-base centers realize their responsibilities for the patient even outside that particular area would also be of help. In any case, the psychological ills of migrancy would be unremitting.

3. Discrimination (++). As in many other solutions, separate services for the migrants would guarantee access to care, but would pose the threat of actual or implied inferiority. If the regional centers were for all persons in a given locale and a sliding scale of fees adopted for non-migrants, and/or the centers were joint-funded with other programs to allow more than just migrants to patronize the center, the threat of discrimination would abate.

If many of the personnel derived from the migrant population, and if administration of the center closely involved a consumer board as the seven 1970 funded projects did, discrimination would be further combated. The avowed aim for quality and comprehensiveness in the centers would provide a sense of pride and self-worth.

Nonetheless, underlying problems of discrimination would remain.

4. Rural Medical Care Capacity (++). By organizing provision of care on a group practice model, by utilizing many non-professional workers, and by seeking to attract physicians from outside the area to fill the positions, the program would be attacking both manpower and organizational problems. If Madison is correct that organized groups are most likely to retain physicians in rural areas (see p. 26), the regional centers would be rather successful. In addition their very existence and prominence might well attract other manpower to the nearby vicinity and encourage still others to go to other rural areas. Despite local successes, the overall input on rural areas would only be slight.

5. Environmental Improvement (++). The capacity to act to improve the environment would be substantial. A permanent large center devoted to health, if it were sufficiently disentangled from the web of local political obligations, would be able to identify environmental problems and press for improvements through a number of channels, primarily legal and political. If the centers had problems with enforcement of improvements, they could at least act to supply relevant information to groups that might have such capability. The centers could also do the job themselves, constructing privies, water systems, and putting up screens.

6. Occupational Hazards (+). The same argument as holds for environmental improvement would hold here. The ultimate possibilities would have

to be tested. Since most work is done upstream, and the program would be weakest there, somewhat less would be expected than with the environment.

7. Malnutrition Alleviation (+). The non-professional personnel of the center, as well as professionals, would be able to intercede on behalf of the migrants with local food stamps or commodity distributors, as well as other official agencies. The main block to better nutrition–money–would be outside the range of services the center could supply.

8. Medical Care Provision (+++). The centers would be well geared to delivering medical care services. The main inhibition to delivering medical care would be the emphasis the center placed on environment, nutrition, or another factor of local choice. Few of the inhibiting factors that would hamper attempts in some of the previous proposals to deliver medical care could hamper this program.

8a. Type of Medical Care Provided (++++). Comprehensive services including preventive and public health care and the full range of primary care services would be provided. Specialist services would be provided on site if demand warranted, or by referral. Hospitalization would not be included in the services offered, a major deficiency necessitated by expense considerations, but the centers would seek to provide hospitalization by non-financial means: enrollment of eligibles in Medicaid, arrangements with public and/or teaching hospitals for limited free admissions, etc.

The quality of care would probably be quite acceptable. Organizational and facility prerequisites for good quality care would be fulfilled. A danger would be that demand for services would mount and initiate the same process that drives private practitioners to cut the quality of their visits. Experience with urban health centers indicates that this tendency can be resisted in centers. The mission, in any case, would remain to deliver in-depth care to the patients, rather than just acute one-time care.

In non-center areas the care would be adjunctive to the major source of care. The quality of those services would be variable, depending on the plan adopted and the locality in question.

Accessibility of services at the centers would be very good, since outreach workers would be active and transportation systems often provided to promote accessibility. Acceptability of services would be expected to be quite high, since the centers would be provided with standard medical center equipment for physicians and patients alike, and since workers in the center would in large part be recruited from the patient population. Staff attitudes would be expected to enhance acceptability.

In sum, the regional health centers would do well on all four standard criteria of the type of medical care provided.

9. Efficiency (++). Theoretically this program should be quite efficient. Many economies of scale should accrue in the center with regard to personnel utilization and facilities.

There should not be a great deal of programmatic red tape, since services would be directly provided. The quality of the services delivered would enhance the efficiency rating. The centers should also be efficient from the patient's point of view, as group practices with adjunctive services are. In addition, the centers should be able to apply for non-migrant health grants, capture Medicaid funds, etc., all of which would act to increase the total production of the operation. The data on the neighborhood health centers, which would be directly applicable, have unfortunately not been clear on the question of efficiency. A major problem has been that so many different services are offered by the centers, the denominator of the calculations of efficiency has been unclear.

On the other hand, long experience with governmental programs indicates that efficiency is not usually a prime asset if bureaucracy is allowed to proliferate. The "bureaucratic factor" would doubtless counteract many of the positive efficiency characteristics.

10. Spillover Effects (+++). There are many opportunities for spillover effects. Migrants would be employed by the centers and trained as aides, outreach workers, and in other capacities. Both jobs and a potential occupation with which to leave the migrant way of life would be provided. In addition, functioning as a community center the regional health centers could provide a nidus for projects aimed at better housing, agricultural cooperatives, or other community projects.

C. Discussion

Of all the proposals, the regional center proposal would provide medical services in the soundest way.

In contrast to the familiar and well-formulated model of group practice medical care with ancillary services, the environmental, occupational, and nutritional components are sketchy at best. With vagueness, however, comes a design for local flexibility, initiative, and potential for action. Unlike the "classical" environmental efforts, the regional health centers would not be beholden to the county commissioners, in all likelihood, and thus a major political impediment to action would be removed. The large size of the project would also be helpful: large projects provide a "critical mass" of employees to consider the problem of their constituents as a whole, since they do not feel themselves so terribly powerless as do small, struggling projects; and large projects provide an organizational flexibility that makes significant action possible.

What the regional health center proposal most clearly lacks is a coherent explanation of environmental problems and a practical agenda to solve them. The proposal is humble in acknowledging that absence, and suggests local flexibility instead.

An attractive example of how a project might structure the environmental and nutritional components would be the following: in years one and two the project would emphasize provision of toilet facilities, clean water, screens, and food for the population; in subsequent years, these activities would be scaled down to maintenance operations, while the medical care component is built up.

Practically, many problems would arise in implementing the regional health center proposal because of its sophistication. The work preparatory to funding a grant would be extremely taxing on both federal officials and local groups. It would be difficult to assemble the proper grantee group and get proper professional and consumer input into planning and then implementation. Recruiting the proper personnel would be difficult, especially for the key post of project administrator. That person would have to be well versed in the intricacies of medical care administration and public health, as well as very understanding of the migrant people. Recruitment of professional medical personnel would be easier, but still difficult. Further problems would come with the continuing functioning of the centers. Federal officials would have to arrange for extensive technical consultation for the projects, to bind the system together and to maintain an esprit de corps that would retard personnel dropout. Significant local political obstacles to be detailed later on would also present problems. The extent of these practical problems should not be underestimated. On the other hand, in 1970 seven projects similar to regional centers were begun and carried through to the present under great time constraints, so it is possible that the problems are overstated.

In many ways this proposal seems like a Christmas tree, with a goodie for every category; some cost estimates will help put it into perspective. In 1970, the seven comprehensive projects were funded at levels just below $400,000 apiece, to serve in excess of 10,000 persons for the six to eight months they were in residence. These were spartan budgets with many frills omitted, and with very little attention to non-medical areas. The more elaborate neighborhood health centers of the Office of Economic Opportunity and the Public Health Service spend two to three times that amount per center to operate year around. If we took an average of $1.2 million per center per year, at the 1975 appropriation level of $25 million, about $20 million could be spent on the centers themselves. About sixteen centers could be operated, then, out of the more than forty counties that would qualify for centers if the term "migrant impact area" were defined as harboring more than 4,000 migrants (not including their families) for six or more months per year. The centers would be able to serve at least 10,000 persons apiece (not all of them migrants), for a total of more than 160,000 persons. This would mean that somewhat less than 20 percent of the migrants would be covered by home-base centers. Since $25 million is probably less than 5 percent of what is necessary to provide comprehensive services to all migrants, stretching it to 20 percent of them would be a fine administrative achievement.

Causal Profile Summary:

(1)	(2)	(3)	(4)	(5)	(6)	(7)	(8)	(8a)	(9)	(10)
0	++	++	++	++	+	+	+++	++++	++	+++

VIII SUMMARY OF CHAPTER 3, AND CONCLUSIONS

Table 3–1 summarizes the evaluative descriptions of the given alternatives. The function of this table is only to delineate the strategic choices made by the various suggested plans; even if the weightings given (from 0 to ++++) were more than general estimates, there would be no general way to judge one strategy preferable to another.

In fact, however, table 3–1 shows that the alternative strategies discussed here are remarkably simple and similar; only alternatives 2 and 8 fail to emphasize medical care to the practical exclusion of anything else. This homogeneity makes column (8a) very important, for it evaluates the different tactics suggested to pursue the medical care strategy, and thus makes a scalar comparison among them. Although each might be used in special situations elucidated in the text above, alternatives 1, 3, 4, 5, 6, and 7 are clearly inferior to alternative 8.

Despite the strategic consensus of most of the alternatives, it should be clear that there is no legitimate underpining for choosing column (8) to emphasize rather than different combinations of columns (1) through (7). The fact that such alternatives are not generated here reflects the task of this chapter and book, which is not to generate numerous alternative strategies, but rather to elucidate in a practical way those that have already been generated, and judge if any "satisfice"—that is, suffice and satisfy.[15] A future task of the MHP should clearly be to generate further alternative proposals and test them theoretically and empirically.

Interestingly, alternatives 8 and 2 represent more than choices of causal elements on which to concentrate; they are really programmatic adaptations to the lack of alternative strategies waiting for evaluation. That is, alternative 8 calls for establishment of large decentralized centers of responsibility for the health of migrants, decentralized enough to be flexible, but aggregated enough to assert a forceful independence. Alternative 2 calls for decentralization to the ultimate degree, to the level of the individual, with the choice set resting on him. Even if we can project where the emphases will lie with these two alternatives, these are simply predictions of the choices of centers not wholly under the control of a centralized program. If one were to add a strong evaluation component with either of these strategies, one would in fact probably be testing various strategic alternatives tried in different localities.

While no definitive choice can be made theoretically between alter-

Table 3-1. Ratings of Policy Alternatives

Program / Criteria*	(1)	(2)	(3)	(4)	(5)	(6)	(7)	(8)	(8a)	(9)	(10)
1. Classical	0	++	+	0	+	0	0	+++	0	0	0
2. Direct cash grant	++++	0	+	0	++	0	++++	+	0	+++	++
3. Insurance	0	+	0	0	0	0	0	++++	0	0	0
4. Referral	0	++	0	0	0	0	+	++++	0	+	0
5. Hospitalization	0	0	0	0	0	0	0	++++	+	0	0
6. Mothers & children	0	++	0	?	0	0	+	++++	?	?	?
7. Mobile clinics	0	+	0	+	0	0	0	++++	0	0	0
8. Regional centers	0	++	++	++	++	+	+	+++	++++	++	+++

*(1) poverty
(2) mobility
(3) discrimination
(4) rural medical capacity
(5) environment
(6) occupational hazards
(7) malnutrition
(8) medical care
(8a) type of medical care
(9) efficiency
(10) spillover

natives 2 and 8, to the extent that medical care should become an important part of the adopted strategy, alternative 8 would be superior. With the other areas such as nutrition and environment, it is not known to what extent aggregation of consumers is necessary and helpful. Medical care, however, has been shown to be unresponsive to market forces, and simply giving migrants money with which they might purchase care will not work. Since the author thinks that medical care provision will inevitably become a major part of the migrant health strategy, he opts for alternative 8. It would also seem plausible that the environmental, occupational, and even nutritional objectives would best be pursued in combined actions, using such federal laws as OSHA and programs such as food stamps as immediate objects of attention; but these are chancier cases, more dependent on the quality of leadership at each individual project than medical care delivery would be.

Chapter Four

Administrative Considerations

This section will consider the changing administrative conditions under which the Migrant Health Program has operated in the past, and will try to draw the implications for future actions. The documentation for this chapter lies chiefly in the personal experience of the author, and a great number of documents in the author's files, not cited in favor of readability.

The discussion first considers the Migrant Health Program and its milieu during the MHP's "classical" period (up until 1969), then the changes that occurred in the program from 1969-1970, with some more fragmentary comments regarding 1971. Finally, the implications of that administrative history for the programmatic changes discussed in Part II are drawn.

I THE MIGRANT HEALTH PROGRAM AND ITS MILIEU, 1962-1969

A. The Federal Government's Role in Health, and the Public Health Services

1. Mission and Operations. The 1960s were years of rapid and great expansion of the federal government's participation in the health sphere. By the end of the decade one could count six major spheres of involvement (some major examples given):

1. Health care financing for needy groups
   *–Medicare, Medicaid
2. Direct provision or grant-financed provision of care for special groups
   –Merchant seamen and others in Public Health Service Hospitals
   –Armed service hospitals, and Veterans Hospitals
   –Indian Health Service

*–Maternal and Child Health, Children and Youth Grants
*–Office of Economic Opportunity Neighborhood Health Centers
*–Neighborhood Mental Health Centers
–Migrant Health Program

3. In-house and Grant financed medical science research
   –National Institution of Health, National Institute of Mental Health
4. Manpower and Facilities Expansion
   –Hill-Burton hospital constructing program
   –research training grants NIH, NIMH
   –other personnel efforts (nurses, etc.)
5. Preventive Medical Services
   –National Center for Disease Control programs, including categorical tuberculosis and venereal disease grants
   –environmental protection programs
6. Medical Care Organizational Change, + Service
   *–Regional Medical Programs
   *–Comprehensive Health Planning
   *–Partnership for Health
   *–OEO Neighborhood Health Centers
   *–Neighborhood Mental Health Centers

Of the above, each starred program was initiated after the Migrant Health Program. It is obvious, then, that the MHP was initiated when federal programs concerned themselves with neither financing nor organizing personal medical services in the country at large.

The pre-MHP programs had three basic ways of operating: grants to and through states, grants directly to researchers, and direct wholly federal operations. By contrast, the programs born after the MHP frequently dealt directly with the country's medical care system, granting money directly to individuals or non-governmental groups as readily as to state governments. The MHP was initiated at the watershed; perhaps for that reason it can be forgiven for being a bit schizophrenic, as this chapter will show it is.

2. PHS Organizational Characteristics. As this marked change in governmental health policies and programs occurred, it was not surprising that the old and traditional Public Health Service should be found less adaptive than some would want. Typical of most long-established organizations, it can aptly be described as a "conserver" organization,[1] dominated by a point of view that assesses a mistake a bigger loss than a triumph is a gain. In other words, the PHS was, with some exceptions, largely content to continue working the traditional programs in the traditional way.

Harold Seidman has cited the Public Health Service as an example in making a more general point:

> Institutional myths and symbols may be worshiped for their own sake long after they have lost their original meaning. Institutional loyalties may be internalized with the result that programmatic goals are displaced, and institutional, professional, or bureaucratic survival and aggrandizement become the overriding objectives. These dysfunctional influences are latent in almost all organizations. Most susceptible are agencies with obsolete, static, or contracting programs or those that are highly in-bred, such as the military, Foreign Service, and Public Health Service.[2]

The PHS is composed of two distinct personnel systems. The Commissioned Corps, operated in a military tradition, composed the original PHS from its inception in 1796, when its original mission was to provide medical care for merchant seamen. Civil Service personnel were added later, and now personnel from each system work side by side indistinguishably. An official commission was set the task of deciding if this anomalous system should be revised, and in 1971 reported to Secretary Elliot Richardson that the Commissioned Corps had not had strong and imaginative personnel for some time, and should be abolished.[3] The Civil Service, while scoring somewhat better, can be characterized with some laudable exceptions in much the same way.

There have been two sources of personnel not fitting the "conserver" designation. First, some officials joined the PHS precisely because they wanted to work with the new programs. Such personnel clustered in the late 1960s in the Division of Medical Care Administration (which dealt with several issues including organizational forms of medical practice, migrant health, and the professional standards of Medicare), Division of Regional Medical Programs, and the Office of Comprehensive Health Planning.

An additional source of personnel not likely to act as "conservers" has been the "two year officers," young physicians and some health administrators serving two years with the PHS as an alternative to the draft. Although most were concentrated in the Indian Health Service dispensing care to Indians on the reservations, a significant number were scattered in the other component parts of the PHS. Many of these individuals come to the PHS with a liberal ideology as well as their desire to avoid the draft, and spurred in part by the realization that they had little to lose in the nature of a PHS career, they frequently proved capable adjuncts to the "non-conservers" of the more permanent officials seeking change, or at least as sources of discontent.

Two more organizational characteristics of the PHS are important for our purposes. First, the PHS has always been fairly well insulated from the outside world. Forming in large part a professional bureaucracy, it has connected closely with state health departments and thence to local health departments in a long chain, with few occasions for interaction with non-professionals. Where such interaction was inevitable, as in the hospitals and Indian Health Service, the use of uniforms and military organization has minimized penetrability. Second, the PHS received its strongest support over the years from the state health departments and the professional organizations in the field, chiefly the American Public Health Association.

In both these characteristics, the PHS is an archetypal model for the structure of a professional bureaucracy with a particular, sectoral interest.[4] It is easy to see, then, how uneasy PHS must have felt as programs calling for interaction with the country at large were thrust upon it.

In this setting, the MHP was a small and unobtrusive program of low salience in the health community, especially after passage of the larger medical care programs.

B. MHP Administrative Organization

Although the legislation permitted the MHP to award grants to a wide variety of groups, in practice the administrators stuck to the traditional and thus non-controversial routes. The state health departments, as we have seen, were given control to some extent of about half of the funds. In return they of course contributed their influence to support the MHP through congressional testimony and other means. So intent was the MHP on dealing with health departments, it even helped create new ones in counties that previously had none. Only in a small number of upstream states were non-governmental groups dealt with.

Inconspicuousness was also nurtured by funding only small projects. The "conserver" tradition dictated that small projects might not make big successes, but they would also be unlikely to get anyone into trouble. Clearly, the MHP acted more like an "old" program than a "new" one.

The personnel administering the MHP in these years was quite stable. The lynch-pin of the group was Helen Johnston, a woman who had started working for the federal government in the Department of Agriculture in the 1930s, and had transferred to the PHS in 1949. She lobbied for a health program for migrant workers for many years, and when one was finally created, it fell primarily to her to assemble the staff. She assigned MHP representatives to the regional offices of HEW in addition to recruiting a central headquarters staff. Major characteristics of the "classical" staff were: (1) virtually none came to the program with a background in primary health care organization; (2) almost all came from non-minority, middle- or lower-middle-class background much more like those of the official personnel in the state and local health departments than those of the ultimate intended recipients of care in 1970, for instance, 190 regional office representatives and only one central staff member spoke Spanish; and (3) although the program did find a number of persons with masters level degrees, the civil service system allotted grade levels of personnel incompatible with high quality in seasoned officials. The MHP, in turn, chose not to recruit young, ambitious persons willing to serve at such levels (as OEO did), but settled for career middle-level civil servants.

Two-year officers assigned to the MHP generally served in the field dispensing medical care, although one did serve as assistant chief of the Migrant Health Branch from 1967 to 1969. He found, however, that his generally moderate suggestions to improve the quality of care in the clinics were rebuffed, even though he was the only physician in the branch.

Constrained by the usual civil service requirements, then, personnel choices were consistent with the traditional pattern of the Public Health Service. The personnel were "conservers" used to dealing with the old type of public health problems (not related to medical care organization, personal services, or the non-governmental sector), and with the interlocking chain of professional agencies. Such choices of personnel were consistent with the requirements of the "classical" MHP program design.

The program's placement in the administrative network also contributed to its inconspicuousness. Although its position shifted rather frequently as reorganizations rent the PHS, it was usually placed as a branch of a rather large division–first the Division of Community Health Services, then the Division of Medical Care Administration, then the Community Health Service (a combination of the former Division of Medical Care Administration and the Office of Comprehensive Health Planning). On the other hand, since the MHP had specific enabling legislation and rather frequent authorization and appropriation hearings, it was more conspicuous than most branches–but it was still only a branch.

The internal mechanics of running the program have been alluded to before. Simply put, there was no detailed program planning, no collection and collation of statistics on a regular basis, and absolutely no evaluation. This point deserves to be emphasized. Every single datum used in this analysis has come from the few congressional hearings available, or from the original project reports the author personally reviewed. Even the data on project size, distribution, services, etc., had to be compiled from scratch (and are subject to some error on the basis of some fragmentary records). Now, it is not uncommon for programs to be deficient in program and project self-evaluation. But it is rather unusual for a program to have no systematic compilation of grantees, amount of awards, and services offered by the grantees on a year-by-year basis. It is unusual, too, for a program to lack even a simple compilation of basic data reported–such as number of patient visits, for example.

Certainly, administrative incompetence could account for some of the deficiencies. Probably more important, however, are the recurrent themes of inconspicuousness and self-protection. To omit project and program evaluation is only half-secure. If one keeps no compiled records at all he ensures much more certainly that he will not be embarrassed even by someone else's evaluation. At the same time, requiring rather detailed (if mostly irrelevant) data from the projects presents a facade of close monitoring. If we suppose, then, that the goal of the MHP's analytic efforts was to maintain programmatic stability and protection from outside attack, far from being incompetent, the analytic efforts were quite skillful.

C. Role of the States

The theme of self-protection and "conserverism," along with preservation of power, recurs in examining the involvement of the state health departments. It was documented earlier how the states were heavily involved. About half the grant funds were directed through the hands of the states, and in 1969 about $900,000, or 11 percent of the available funds, went directly to the states for consultation and related non-service activities.

The official rationale for the consultation projects was the need for continued project surveillance and assistance in addition to direct PHS activities, the need for inter-project coordination, and the need for interstate coordination. A latent motive must have been that the MHP was very anxious to hold to the traditional PHS approach, with the assurance of support and insulation from outside influences that such channels provided.

In fact, it turned out that the state health departments did provide a good deal of legislative support, as can be traced in all the congressional hearings. More problematical has been the direct contribution of the state health departments to the program. The quality of the local projects certainly offers no positive indications of state assistance. This is not surprising, for the same kind of personnel who inhabit the federal level are encountered at the state level—no physicians, no persons knowledgeable about medical care organization, "conservers," etc. Much like the federal officials, they were content to serve primarily as grants managers. The coordinating role for states was from the start a chimera. It makes no sense to facilitate transfer of a patient from one project to another, if neither does a proper job of delivering medical care. In sum, little programmatic aid was forthcoming from the state health departments.

Three anecdotes characterize the role of the states more concretely. The first incident indicates that the "classical" administration was well aware and accepted the fact that the state projects were funded for political-administrative and not programmatic reasons. Early in 1969, just following the MHP reorganization to be described shortly, some efforts were contemplated at headquarters to make the state-level projects "pull their weight." The state health department project in Texas was then the case in point. Usually site visits following up the periodic project review sessions were made by PHS teams of central and regional personnel, with at most nominal participation by the states. It was suggested that the Texas project itself be called upon to make some of these visits. This suggestion was strongly opposed by the former chief of the Migrant Health Branch, Miss Johnston, on the grounds that the state project was clearly "incompetent," although her program had been awarding grants to that project unquestioningly for many years. In the context of discussion it was quite clear that she meant what she said quite literally, and had felt it necessary to sacrifice money for such a project in order to receive in return the traditional favorable testimony, and avoid opposition from the state health officer before the congressional committees.

An example from Florida illustrates the state health department's view of its function and powers. For years the state-level project had been staffed primarily by a former sanitarian whose main function was visiting local projects for "liaison" purposes. In the midst of the 1969–70 MHP program changes, the state was offered a chance to improve its project by employing a full-time physician, for the express purpose of using the newly prepared Guidelines as an instrument for qualitative project improvements. Accepting the new position, the health department promptly assigned a near-retirement physician from another of its branches; the PHS regional representative had known the state was looking for a place to let this elderly man finish his service, and although scandalized, he felt the MHP could do little about the appointment. Adding injury to insult, the newly appointed physician promptly went to the local projects with the message that in his view the Guidelines should be ignored. More powerful than most, this state health department was quite capable of preserving its power and buffering the local projects from the erratic winds of the federal government, and could even turn the neat bureaucratic trick of increasing the resources while doing it.

California had one of the most progressive state health departments in the nation, and its migrant health effort was led by a dynamic, even inspirational Chicano social worker. In contradistinction to other state level projects, California constantly urged the local projects to improve their efforts, offered helpful consultations in the field of nursing, and compiled statistics that exceeded by far anything the national program could muster. Despite the programmatic differences, when push came to shove, California acted much like Florida.

In view of the promising record of the California state project the MHP federal administrators seeking change in 1970 sought to coopt it into aiding the change efforts. The project personnel were ambivalent, feeling some change was necessary, but doubtful of their own ability to carry it out, and reluctant to cede their prerogatives to let anyone else carry it out. They vacillated, but in the end tried to block several of the new projects and to recoup their lost prerogatives. These efforts were unsuccessful, however, because, first, inexperienced in fighting against the Feds, they could not develop a coherent political strategy and stick to it, and second, they were Democrats serving in the Reagan administration and thus had trouble at arriving at common grounds with top Department of Public Health officials.

In summary, the state-level projects took a major investment of the MHP's resources, and yielded in return mostly political and structural benefits. The states lent congressional and professional support to the program, provided a tradition of arrangements comforting to the MHP administrators, and provided a buffer between the PHS and local projects, thus insulating the MHP even further from possible external jolts.

D. The Role of County Health Departments

As the state health departments were treated in the old tradition, so too were county health departments viewed as the "natural" recipients for local PHS grants. This view was strengthened by the fact that pioneering work was done in migrant health in two unusual health departments in Palm Beach, Florida, and Fresno, California. Just as the PHS and state health departments had little or no experience with primary health care organization, so too with the local health departments. Their usual functions consisted of environmental health inspection in the community, categorical clinics and investigatory functions for infectious diseases such as tuberculosis, venereal diseases, and the immunizable diseases, and occasionally some small forays into well-baby clinics of family planning clinics.

The MHP required these county health departments to change their function markedly. Several organizational factors made such change difficult. First of all, the professional capabilities of the local health departments in America have not been of the highest. The post of County Health Officer is not very prestigious, and the professional quality of men filling the post is often mediocre. The public health nurses, on the other hand, tend to stand much higher in their profession, and are often rather aggressive and able, within the limits of the culturally prescribed female and nursing roles. In fact, the informal leadership of migrant health projects has often rested with a nurse.[5] The rest of the staff tends to be generally undistinguished. None has training or experience in the organization of primary medical care, since their jobs have always been construed quite differently.

With the exception of some of the nurses, most of the county health department personnel are "conserver" in type. There are few if any personal advancements to be made, and virtue lies in avoiding mistakes or failures.

The question arises, then, what would induce such an organization to apply for and accept a migrant grant? One answer would be the possibility of increasing the health department budget and number of personnel, if the risks could be kept down, plus the incentive of avoiding embarrassment and stigmatization as incompetent if such grants should be available and desired by some parts of the community, and the health department were to be found not to have secured one. In addition, the fact that the PHS and state health departments were involved would make for a sense of security, and a sense that this was a job that the local health departments were now supposed to do. Finally, motivation comes from an idealism that brought many—once again, especially the nurses—into the field of public health. Not infrequently, their feelings of wanting to help the poor with no thought of personal advancement is sincere and persistent.

Administratively, the county health department answers to two bosses, one up the county government chain, and one up the public health chain. The former can set impenetrable limits beyond which the health department cannot go, and it can also intervene directly. The latter's influence is not so direct, but controlling a great deal of the grant resources as it does, it is able to be quite effective in molding the actions of the local health departments.

Local government is by definition in the hands of the political establishment. In the rural areas, as elsewhere, the poor do not form part of that establishment. While it is clear the establishment forces are not necessarily opposed to migrant health, some limitations are immediately set. For instance, the environmental issue cannot be pressed, since this would implicate the establishment. The health effort must include measures that decrease the possibility of migrants' harboring diseases that might spread to the constituency of the office holders—i.e., there must be a focus on infectious disease and immunizations, no matter what. Ideologically, a limit is set on the health department doing "too much" for the migrant. Any infringement, real or imagined, on the realm of the private practitioner is also likely to be squelched.

A second limit placed on health departments has to do with employment practices. Firstly, the county government can use its influence to procure jobs for its protégés, as long as they meet the requirements of the merit system. Secondly, the prescribed adherence to the merit system can block the creation of non-standard jobs (e.g. health aides with significant duties), and can prescribe sub-poverty level salaries for the types of jobs migrants are likely to qualify for.

The county health departments' other masters, the Public Health Service and the state health departments, are professional, "conserver" organizations; both are likely to insist on the proper qualifications for all employees. Both are likely to encourage the health department to keep a "low profile" and not risk much of a venture into new areas. All three organizations are likely to reinforce one another in a devotion to "professional standards," which means a turning inward, rather than a turning outward to the community. It should also mean truly rigorous standards, and good medical care, but in medical care, Chapter 2 has shown that such is not the case. The explanation lies in adherence to an inappropriate set of professional standards, standards dealing with public health services, not personal health services.

The county health departments ran their projects making a few changes in their regular operating philosophies and procedures as possible. In light of the above administrative considerations, such action does not seem unusual.

E. Role of the Project Review Committee

As many programs have done, the MHP used the Surgeon General's general authority to establish an external review committee, called the Migrant Health Project Review Committee (MHPRC). The usual functions of such committees are to lend political support and professional guidance to the program. The MHPRC gave little professional guidance, but did offer some political support.

The MHPRC was rather faithful in representing the constituency of the MHP. A recent list of members includes: a Catholic sister, a hospital administrator from New Mexico; a health educator from the University of Minnesota; a berry grower from the state of Washington; the director of Special Health Services of the Colorado State Health Department; an MHP project director from the University of Puerto Rico; a professor of sociology from Houston; a physician from Fresno, California, who is chairman of the AMA council on Rural Health; the South Florida representative of the Florida Board of Health; a social worker from New Orleans; and a member of the Migrant Ministry from Texas. A member of the United Farm Workers Organizing Committee was formerly included at the direction of the top echelons of HEW, but reportedly declined to attend meetings. No one was chosen for the MHPRC who would have been likely to cause controversy. No member was militant, none was a migrant, and none a specialist in medical care organization. None was even particularly distinguished within his field of expertise.

The triannual meetings were marked by an absence of controversy as all projects were reviewed and approved, some wholeheartedly, some with reservations. All projects were regarded warmly rather than critically, and as the project longevity figures show, projects were virtually never discontinued. With no specific standards against which to judge the projects, the little hard information, meaningful decisions were difficult to come by. The basic preconceptions of the program—sponsorship, size of grants, etc.—were never questioned at these meetings. In line with the general propensity of the MHP, one would be hard-pressed to choose a "safer" panel.

F. Summary

The MHP was initiated just before the federal government became involved in the delivery of personal health services to civilian Americans to a large extent, and just before the PHS broke off its practice of making all service grants through state health departments. The PHS during these years was a basically "conserver" organization, with two sources of "non-conserver" personnel: medical care administration experts interested in personal health service programs, and "two-year" PHS officers. The PHS, as a professional organization, was well insulated from outside influences, and derived major support from professional agencies and organizations. Even at the beginning and to a larger extent later on, the MHP assumed a position of low salience and visibility in the medical care world.

The MHP was administered in a very traditional way, although the law was flexible. Grants were made predominantly to traditional PHS grant recipients, and the small size of grants further protected the administrators. The administrative personnel chosen had no previous experience with primary care organization, were white middle-class persons themselves, and had Civil Service ratings incompatible with highly developed competence in officials of their age.

The "two-year" officers were employed in the field delivering medical care. The Migrant Health Branch remained a small branch in a large PHS division. Internally, there was little reliance placed on planning or evaluation, thus enhancing the protection of the Migrant Health Branch.

Although the state health departments received 11 percent of MHP funds for administrative and consultative duties, the organizational and political support they rendered was much more impressive than their programmatic support. The states were jealous of their powers, and often buffered the local projects from PHS attempts to change them.

The county health departments became grantees out of tradition, although they had no relevant experience or expertise in primary medical care, and although their organizational characteristics made changes difficult for them. Their reasons for wanting MHP grants included increases in their budget and personnel complement, protection from community pressure, security in being associated with the state health departments and the PHS, and idealism. Structural organizational requirements for the county health departments came from both county governments and public health authorities. The former set limits on possible infringement on established power in personal medical care and environmental control, enforced more general county norms, and in addition influenced employment practices for projects to favor permanent county residents and discourage migrants. The public health authorities for their part supported employment according to rigid professional standards, encouraged the projects to retain a "low profile," and encouraged adherence to standards inappropriate for the delivery of primary medical care.

The Migrant Health Project Review Committee contained representatives of groups supporting the MHP, looked fondly and permissively on the MHP projects, and conducted little substantive review of program or projects.

II MIGRANT HEALTH PROGRAM CHANGES, 1969–1970

In January 1969 a reorganization broke up the encapsulated MHP administration and exposed it to the forces that had changed the PHS in the six years since the MHP's inception. After that, attempts at programmatic change came quickly.

A. Reorganization

The Division of Medical Care Administration, which contained the Migrant Health Branch, was constructed to perform the professional services required by Medicare, passed in 1965. This division increasingly became a center for specialists in medical care organization. In late 1968 the Office of Comprehensive Health Planning left its direct attachment to the Surgeon General's office and was merged with DMCA, creating the Community Health Service (CHS). With the office of Comprehensive Health Planning came responsibility for administering section 314(e) of the Public Health Service Act, the most aggressive of the new PHS programs. Under its authority grants for neighborhood health centers (NHC) stressing consumer participation in administration were awarded.

The Division of Health Care Services composed a major part of CHS; its task was to administer 314(e), the Migrant Health Program, and the Appalachian Health Program. Since the latter was run chiefly by the Appalachian Regional Commission, the division's major programs were 314(e) and the MHP. In a move calculated to open up the MHP to new ideas and new people, the division was organized along functional lines—one branch responsible for initiation of new projects, one concerned with proper development of already established projects, one with technical assistance resource development, and one for program review and record keeping. Each branch was thus to handle both MHP and 314(e) grants. Members of the abolished Migrant Health Branch were scattered to the new functional branches and the former chief of the Migrant Health Branch was made coordinator for Migrant and Rural Health, reporting directly to the division director and with no line authority.

In this radically changed situation, a great deal of de facto headquarters programmatic control of the MHP was exercised for fourteen or sixteen months by a gradually evolving and changing small group of "two-year" physicians (and some "two-year" men extending their stay), the initiator and former administrator of the Alviso, California, Neighborhood Health Center (at the time the best Chicano health center in the country, with full community control), and a middle-aged medical care organization specialist who was formerly a key member of the OEO health team.[a]

Somewhat later, the California regional office was reorganized in a similar way; that office then consisted of a "two-year" physician, a "two-year" medical care organization specialist, the regional migrant health representative, and two medical care organization specialists slightly senior to the "two-year" men.

It happened that the "two-year" men at headquarters and in California, while of course in the PHS to avoid the draft, had sought to be placed in just such roles because of the interest and prior experience with medical care programs and social problems.

All these people were far from "conservers," but could better be described as "climbers" (again Anthony Downs' term).[6] They had everything to gain from change and little to lose. The "two-year" men would soon be out of the PHS, probably, and thus were not subject to career-type sanctions. The physicians in particular had a multitude of options. They also had reputations to make in the field, and political and social philosophies to express.

The more permanent officials also had strong motivations for change. The former Alviso director deliberately sought to associate himself with a pro-

[a]The principal physicians were the author and James M. Perrin, the former Alviso director was Thomas V. Uridel, and the former OEO employee was John Frankel.

gram that was concerned with migrants, and one where change to the Alviso way of thinking was a real possibility. Not really a career type, he viewed himself as with the government temporarily, to see what it was like, and what changes in favor of social justice could be made within its confines. The other officials were young and on the way up, with progressive social ideas, and with the possibility of progressing professionally, if not in the PHS, then elsewhere. The former OEO official was no longer young, but had a passionate belief in social justice and the OEO type of operation. Downs would probably classify him as a "statesman" rather than a "climber."

> Although all officials occasionally behave like statesmen, consistent statesman like behavior in bureaus is extremely rare. It is most likely to be encountered either at the very lowest or the very highest levels. Statesmen are found at the lowest levels because men who enter bureaus and consistently evidence statesmanlike behavior are rarely promoted.[7]

Four more officials should be discussed. First, the newly appointed division director, although not a strong leader, was a professional researcher with some standing in the field of medical care organization. Any professional advances made in his division would be a feather in his professional cap. Any failures would be written off by the profession as a negative experiment—a not uncommon occurrence. Possibilities of promotion within the PHS were also present for him. He was, therefore, in favor of change, although he was anxious to hedge his bet by making no explicit alliances with—nor granting much formal authority to—the aforementioned change-oriented group. Along with most others, he was really more interested in the newer, larger, and more conspicuous 314(e) program than with the MHP.

The director and deputy director of the Community Health Service were cut more from the "conserver" mold, but not completely so. They tended to act as mediators between the contending factions, as the Coordinator for Rural and Migrant Affairs (the former Migrant Health Branch chief) led a rear guard fight against changing the MHP. They, too, had most of their attention riveted on 314(e), which they had to fight to keep in their organization.

Finally, the administrator of the Health Services and Mental Health Administration, to whom the CHS director reported, was a recently appointed young activist transfer from OEO, ideologically close to the group seeking change, but beset by severe problems of his own (politically, as a Kennedy Democrat serving in the Nixon administration, and administratively, in having to contend with his conserver subordinates), which were to lead to his dismissal in the spring of 1970. He was particularly close to his old OEO colleague, now working with the MHP, and the former Alviso director, whom he (the administrator) had personally recruited to the PHS.

These, then, were the preconditions for programmatic change—a massive headquarters shift of responsibility to change-oriented personnel, and change in the California regional office.

B. Events of Change

1. The Guidelines. Two major battles were fought over change; the first was over the issue of project Guidelines. The "change-agent" group started to develop the Guidelines in 1969 with the intent of defining specific, minimal criteria for migrant health projects, to ensure that an effective and efficient system was set up with good quality medical care, progressive program administration, and strong migrant input, much in the NHC mold. Once developed, the Guidelines would be a useful tool to build new projects and change or discontinue old ones.

Development of the Guidelines started in the spring of 1969 and continued desultorily throughout the period we are discussing. The change from the regional MHP representatives by frequent consultation, although the relationship was clearly one-sided. The regional representatives were called in several times in a group to comment on successive drafts of the document; to assure them that the medical care requirements of the Guidelines were solidly based, the section detailing medical care standards was developed in meetings between practicing project physicians (selected by the regional representatives), the physicians from MHP headquarters, and the regional representatives themselves. Fewer such efforts were made in developing other sections, but there was much discussion.

The regional representatives, although at first wary of changes, came to the point of actually calling for issuance of the Guidelines in the fall of 1969. If there were to be programmatic changes, they would be happy to have a clear document to work from. In late 1969 and early 1970, many copies of the then current draft were circulated unofficially to state health departments and some local projects. The comments and reactions provoked were mixed. Further refining of the document by the central staff, and an inability to move the document through the uncertain channels towards official approval, combined to delay official issuance.

In the early 1970 HEW decided to decentralize the MHP administration to the regional offices; this move upset the slow but steady progress of the Guidelines. Decentralization was not based on anything specific to the MHP, but was rather part of the general strategy of the new administration in HEW to decentralize. A committee was appointed to effect the change; the division director appointed members of the "classical" program to head the committee, and the committee declared that the Guidelines fell into their purview.

Given this chance, the former Migrant Health Branch chief quickly rallied her forces to produce a rival set of Guidelines, based on the original but considerably watered down. With two sets now in existence, approval possibilities for either set quickly deteriorated, and it was fully one year later that a compromise set was set up for approval through channels. Finally, a condensed version was approved as official regulations.

From the start the Guidelines had significant impact. They were rather widely circulated and clearly painted an image of a changing program. They also focused attention on the subjects most important to the "change-agents": project sponsorship, quality of care, and mode of organization.

Another result of the Guidelines was that they crystallized the federal administrators into two camps, one offensive and one defensive, with some permanent and some "swing" member in each. The strategy of attempted cooption of the regional representatives by the "change-agents" tended to minimize their opposition to the new ideas, and to highlight them as a significant source of power. Their relatively low rank, character, and "conserver" incentives, however, made the regional representatives reluctant to act as arbiters in the conflict at headquarters. They sought rather to cover their bets in both camps, although in general preferring the "classical" camp. Significantly, personal relationships between the regional representatives and change-group, although not close and clearly potentially quite antagonistic, were strained as little as possible by that strategy.

All this, despite the impact of the "change-agents," would have constituted successful resistance to change, had it not been for the second major issue.

2. The New Projects. The second major issue came to the fore in early 1970, just as the Guidelines issue was at a late peak. The HEW budget for the fiscal year was passed with only about four months remaining before all the money had to be obligated. For reasons totally divorced from the internal controversies we have been considering here (as far as we know), the MHP received a large increase in appropriation, from $8 million to $15 million. Although both of the contending factors in the MHP had assured the Bureau of the Budget and all others concerned that all the new money could be spent expeditiously on projects already planned, in fact the "change-agent" faction wanted to accept the new money as a challenge to new programming, realizing that most of the "old money" was essentially immobile because of the usual political difficulties in reallocating funds. The "classical faction," on the other hand, felt that with a short lead time most of the new money would have to be spent on their old projects, and certain new projects of the old type waiting in the wings. The program's credibility with the Congress and Bureau of the Budget would be undermined were it to seek to impede allocation of the new funds; both factions hoped to capitalize on the short lead time in the meantime.

The division director was convinced to keep the new money largely separate from the old, and base the priorities for new project funding on the latest draft of the Guidelines. The short lead time, the on-going process of decentralization, and staff controversy combined to make the situation distinctly unusual. Joint action by regional and central staff pressed by the regional representatives, was therefore adopted. A meeting of both central and regional MHP staff initiated the programming efforts, and such a meeting was used to achieve agreement on the final funding decisions. In the meanwhile, members of the central staff—some "change-agents," some old line MHP—were assigned one to each regional office for the purpose of new programming. Although the idea was that only the best projects would be funded, all concerned realized that some sort of proportional regional allocation would have to be made. In the end, about half of the new money went for old-style projects, and about half for new style ones.

It is useful to summarize the results region by region. The California Regional Office sat in the "change-agent" camp, and even before the new money arrived had made contact with two consumer groups in the Central Valley that would be potential grantees. Subsequent work in conjunction with the headquarters "change-agents" and the California Rural Legal Assistance program turned up two other West Coast consumer groups as potential grantees. The choice was made to confer with and conciliate the local medical groups only to the extent of allowing them to cooperate and enter the programs voluntarily, but allowing them as little chance to act negatively as possible. The short interval between grant writing and grant award contributed to success in bypassing hostile groups. Since the California regional office, their central office consultant, and the consultant they employed from the SALUD health center, were quite sophisticated in primary care organization, many progressive medical care features were incorporated in the grants. The regional officials maintained the confidence of their grantees in all cases. Professional recruitment of project directors and physicians was handled jointly by grantees and regional office, with good success. Each of the four grants was funded at an initial level of about $400,000.

In the Denver regional office programming was handled by a "two-year" man quite current on all relevant concepts and favorable to the "change-agent" ideas. Working in concert with a group formerly associated with the Denver neighborhood health center complex, and a "change-agent" from headquarters, he stimulated creation and funding of a project in the Weld County area, over the strenuous objection of the county health department, and subsequently the state health department, both of whom would of course have preferred to see the funding come their way. The biggest problem in this generally progressive project appeared to be consumer involvement, since there was apparently no preexisting consumer organization in the area.

The Atlanta regional office chose Florida as their target area. There were some progressive influences in the regional office, but the regional representative was rather old line. The assignee from headquarters was one of the more aggressive "two-year" men. In competition between two possible centers, one sponsored solely by a university, the other a cooperative venture of a migrant consumer group, a university medical school, and a health planning agency, the second center was chosen chiefly because of the influence of the "two-year" man. The primary care emphasis of the program was insured by reliance on the sophisticated Department of Family Medicine in the medical school for the technical planning. A strong voice for the migrants was nurtured by placing a consumer majority on the governing board and seeking to connect its operations somewhat with the aforementioned organized migrants. Broad provider support was sought from the medical society, the hospitals, and other groups, although the health department was extremely reluctant to lend its blessing or support. It had been the original inclination of the Atlanta regional representative to rely primarily on the health department for the program; enlistment of the other groups was on the initiative of the "two-year" man, and caused the regional representative some anguish.

In Upper New York State a program was mounted on a provider base—the local health planning group, the former migrant project, and a hospital. The federal representatives were the unreconstructed New York regional office, and an eager but politically inexperienced "two-year" man from headquarters. While technically rather sound, the project never really involved the consumers. Such upstream areas are of course more difficult for consumer organizations, and the undoubted sincerity of some of the project people was reflected in an action one year after funding, when three of them were suspended for trying to press suit against the State of New York for allegedly improperly certifying certain camps. Their suspension attests to the essential weakness of their position.

The final case of a project that might qualify as a "new look" project was in Michigan, where a relatively enlightened health officer worked to establish a large project centered on primary care, but with no consumer voice. This project had been in the planning stage for at least a year, and was handled on the federal side by a member of the "classical" MHP team who was sympathetic to the primary care concept. The project was regionally based, had several primary care dispensing points and a referral system, and did not involve consumers in operations. Technically, its organization seems midway between the classical pattern and the new projects just described.

About half the new money was spent for projects in a more traditional mold. The Northeast region with the regional office in Boston hosts few migrants, but traditionally provided some services for those coming into the region. This low priority issue (from the regional office's point of view) was handled primarily by a young "two-year" health services administrator with guidance from the "change-agents" in headquarters. The state governmental agency in charge of the program was also amenable to change and programmed some money accordingly to "buy into" some functioning group practices in behalf of their clients. Although a project of small scale, this case does represent an attempt to find new solutions.

The Chicago-based region represents a sort of transition situation, for although they were responsible for programming the large comprehensive project in Michigan, the main initiative for that project came from the health department in Benton Harbor. The remainder of the regional efforts, although sincerely conceived by that region to embody the new approach, in fact betrayed a lack of understanding of what it entailed. The headquarters representative, although clearly of higher caliber than the regional representative, came from the same background—a veteran of the "classical" program, he was now trying to form new habits and learn new concepts. Accordingly, the old stand-by grantee, the Ohio State Health Department, was programmed to receive a large grant, instead of the small grants of the past. Exactly what would be done with the grant, however, was far from clear at the time of the grant submittal. Eventually, a somewhat more intensive application of the traditional techniques resulted.

Region VI, based in Kansas City, seemed to be oblivious to the changes taking place. The regional representative there was a soon-to-retire elderly lady of doubtful health, there were rather few migrants in the area, and the MHP was of rather low salience to the regional office. Several small grants to health departments resulted from that region's efforts at programming. The headquarters temporary helper in the region was also clearly "classical," and lent support for these traditional efforts.

Region III, based in Charlottesville, Virginia, and including the large home-base area of Puerto Rico, had as their Migrant Health representative a man of about sixty years of age who had been in the Public Health Service since 1935, and had worked in the venereal disease program for twenty-five years before becoming a Migrant Health Regional Representative in 1964. Clearly hostile to change in operations in the program, this official utilized rather familiar bureaucratic ploys to avoid overt hostilities but still to keep his region's projects traditional. He undercut some active but sporadic attempts by central headquarters to stimulate a new type program in Puerto Rico, and programmed a new one in another area of the island, using the university and health department as grantees. Although the program was not greatly different from the usual ones, the regional representative increased the size of the grant application and used new terminology for traditional project activities to assume the trappings of change without the substance. This region was not covered by a headquarters representative.

Finally, the Dallas, Texas, regional office was responsible for covering the largest center of migrants in the country—the Lower Rio Grande Valley. There were two MHP regional representatives in this office, both close to forty years of age, both former venereal disease investigators. Both were reluctant to make programmatic changes, and adopted tactics that, although more straightforward than those of the regional representative from Region III, still were designed to retard the proposed programmatic changes. To aid them in the new programming effort two representatives were sent from headquarters, one an unreconstructed "classical" team member and the other a "two-year" physician just nine months in the PHS, but completely familiar with the concepts of comprehensive primary health care. Despite the capabilities and influence of the latter, the will of the regional office was pervasive, and attempts at new style projects were weak.

Two incidents in Texas are illustrative of the peculiar dilemmas of Texas. The Lower Rio Grande Valley has the largest collection of migrant workers for the longest time each year in the country. For some years grants had been awarded to the four counties in question, all run by the same health officer, a retired air force medical officer. The projects were recognized as grossly inadequate—in their mode of operation as well as scope—by the regional office itself. Before the new money became available, one of the "two-year" headquarters physicians had tried to cultivate a grant application from a migrant organization in the Valley. Before sufficient progress could be made, the regional office insisted this "two-year" man not return to the Valley, because he was "not coordinating sufficiently" with the regional office.

So it was another "two-year" man who was sent to help Texas develop new proposals. He was anxious to continue the broken-off negotiations with the increasingly suspicious Chicano group, but was held on a very tight rein by the regional office, and soon was instructed to spend most of his efforts elsewhere. The regional representatives made no efforts to get this Chicano group and the health department to cooperate. They also ignored the overtures of the local medical society, whose new president had reversed the policy of his predecessors by declaring himself in favor of federal grants, and eager to cooperate with them. Finally, the regional representatives also failed to provide any consultation with the development of the grant applications.

The result, then was predictable. Separate grant proposals came in from the Chicano group (using a Catholic sisters' group as a funding agent) and the health department, neither involving the Valley physicians, and both of poor technical quality. A moderate sized grant was subsequently awarded to the regional office's preferred grantee, the health department, and little change in project operations was noted. A year later the migrant advocate grant was funded, suggesting the bureaucratic strife itself determined much of the regional office actions, but lack of adequate organizational direction has proved a persistent problem.

The other incident illustrates the difficulties of local politics in Texas. The regional office had located a young osteopath in Mathis, Texas, who was accustomed to giving a great deal of service to the local poor community, and who had an unorthodox life style as well. After word got out that he was soon to receive a grant to help him care for more migrants, he was arrested for drunkenness by the local authorities, and subsequently shot and killed while allegedly trying to escape. [8] While the local atmosphere is not always so stark as in Mathis, it is clear that the regional office would find difficulties championing the cause of the poor in an aggressive manner.

Some generalizations from these region-by-region experiences can be made. First, it did prove possible in the short time of only several months to program many projects that met the requirements of the Guidelines, which basically sought to define the type of project called a Regional Health Center in this report. The projects have not been well evaluated, but were seen as successful as the comparable OEO centers. The conclusion seems warranted that programming through non-health directed groups can be successful; indeed, it seems better to program through groups that have no health "template," than through health departments that have misleading ones. Whereas the health departments steadfastly resisted change of concepts, the other groups were much more amenable to technical direction.

The problem of professional recruitment has also been shown to be somewhat easier to solve, at this non-extensive level of demand and with this short time frame, than would have been predicted. Such is the case for physicians as well as project directors, quality as well as quantity. One cannot distinguish the effectiveness of the different methods used—personnel recruiting outside the local area for the West Coast projects, local recruiting elsewhere. The competitive salaries allowed have probably had an important bearing on the success of the efforts. Recruitment should not be viewed as a serious short-run problem for starting new centers.

One must despair of drawing conclusions regarding the proper formula for producing a successfully designed and executed project. Table 4–1, however, provides a useful summary of the new programming experience, and can serve as the basis for some tentative judgments.

It seems that a strong federal hand to help design the project is necessary at some point. This conclusion is particularly understandable when we are talking about projects emanating from non-health groups. In Table 4–1 it is evident that in Regions III and VI, where there was no such federal presence, projects judged "–,–" in the quality columns emerged. These regions are both mainly upstream regions, with the exception of Puerto Rico in Region III, but other upstream areas were able to do better. Regions V and II almost conform to the same pattern.

At the other end of the spectrum, where both headquarters assignee and regional office were strong—Regions VIII and IX—the projects emerged as "+, +" quality projects. Region I nearly conforms to that pattern; the explanation for the problem with migrant input is to be found in its upstream location.

Regions IV and VII, then, are the two regions where there were direct conflicts between the philosophies of the headquarters representative and the regional offices. In the case of Region IV, headquarters won, in the case of

Table 4-1. Summary of Programming Experiences

					Project Quality	
(1)	*(2)*	*(3)*	*(4)*	*(5)*	*(6)*	*(7)*
Region Number and Headquarters	*Headquarters Assignee Orientation*	*Regional Office Personnel Orientation*	*Location*	*Consumer Group Presence*	*Technical Medical Quality*	*Migrant Input*
I Boston	none	+	U	– ?	+	–
II New York	±	–	U	– ?	±	–
III Charlottesville	none	–	U-H	– ?	–	–
IV Atlanta	+	–	H	+	+	+
V Chicago	±	–	U	+	±	–
VI Kansas City	–	–	U	– ?	–	–
VII Dallas	+	–	H	+	–	–
VIII Denver	+	+	U	– ?	+	+
IX San Francisco	+	+	H-U	+	+	+

Symbol explanation:

(a) columns (2) and (3)–estimates of orientation of personnel on basis of knowledge of and adherence to objectives of the "change-agent" group: + indicates adherence, – non adherence. Hdq. assignee for regions II and V judged ± because region II's lacked experience with the program, and region V's adherence can only be judged questionably.

(b) column (4)–U = upstream; H = home base

(c) column (5)–since most regions did not search for consumer groups, one cannot be sure whether any exist or not.

(d) column (6)–+ indicates general adherence to the Guidelines in the projects designed. Regions II's and V's major projects are deviant in a substantial number of areas.

(e) column (7)–+ indicates clear designation of migrant input into projects, not a prediction of whether or not the input will eventuate and be effective.

Region VII, the regional office won. The pertinent factors seem to have been that regional office VII was rather implacably opposed to change, while regional office IV was not so opposed at first (a change in regional program director later solidified the opposition to change). Secondly, the headquarters representative to Region IV had more prestige than the one to Region VII. Thirdly, special circumstances in Dade County in Florida, including a progressive nearby medical school and a strong group of migrant advocates as well as a strong migrant leader, enabled the headquarters representative to form a coalition that proved strong enough to carry the day. The local circumstances in Texas were far more difficult.

In the future it would seem that federal strength should lie at least in the regional offices, where the day-to-day nurturing must go on, and where the information flow to headquarters can be most often controlled. The present decentralized administration strengthens this tentative conclusion.

Project location must also be considered. The four regions with home-base areas have remarkably contrasting program design scores: two are "+, +" and two are "–,–." The upstream areas are likewise variable. One can say this, however: given that a project receives a score of + or ± for technical design (Regions I, II, IV, V, VIII, IX), if it is an upstream project it is likely to receive a – score for migrant input (3 of 4), but if it is homebase, it is likely to receive a + score for migrant input (2 of 2). There is an aberrance in Region VIII, but the scores are given only for project design, not for effectuation. That the Region VIII project can bring about effective consumer participation is problematical. An exception not reflected in the figures occurs in Region IX. Their project in the Yakima Valley of Washington is upstream, but it is based on a cooperative society of "settled-out" migrants, and is therefore quite strong with consumer input, although there are many potential conflicts present.

The resulting conclusion relating project design and location is, unsurprisingly, that home-base projects are more likely to have strong consumer participation than upstream projects.

C. Summary

The multiple reorganizations that gripped the PHS during its change of mission in the 1960s hit the MHP in 1969, shattering its former isolation. The MHP was administered side by side with 314(e), which sponsored neighborhood health centers; the two types of non-conserver personnel found in the PHS, "two-year" officers and medical care organization experts, started to administer the MHP; the two types of non-conserver personnel found in the PHS, "two-year" officers and medical care organization experts, started to administer the MHP; one regional office was fully reorganized along the same lines, the two others assigned "two-year" officers to the MHP; and HSMHA officials were installed who supported change in the MHP, although it was of low salience to them.

The first change event was an attempt by the "change-agents" to institute a set of project guidelines to serve as the basis for new project building and old project changing. Their strategy involved cooption of the MHP regional representatives, resistance came from the "classical" MHP forces, and the result was an atmosphere of change and conflict, little immediate substantial change, but eventual approval of many of the Guideline items as official regulations.

The second change event centered around $6.8 million of project funds appropriated to the MHP with only several months available for programming. Programming was accomplished in regional office–central office teams. Half the money wound up devoted to new style projects, half to old style projects. It was found that new style projects could be programmed quickly and well, that it was advantageous to deal with groups who did not have the wrong design ideas to begin with, and that recruitment of manpower proved no immediate obstacle. Where both central and regional federal officials were strong, strong project proposals resulted, by the terms of the Guidelines; where both were weak, so were the projects. In mixed situations, the results were variable. Significant migrant input was more likely in the home-base areas.

III MIGRANT HEALTH PROGRAM REGROUPING, 1970–71

The change in personnel that followed the new programming effort took place as rapidly as had the initial reorganization that brought the "change-agents" in the first place. Most of the major "change-agents" left quickly. The former OEO official had a heart attack even before the programming and was induced to retire. The major headquarters "two-year" man left in July as his term of service ended; his choice not to remain on the job was made firm by the apparent lack of possibilities for much more progress, and the appearance of a reaction against change in the upper echelons at headquarters.

The division director was replaced even before the grants were awarded. The HSMHA administrator himself was ousted in a political move of the Republican HEW Administration to rid themselves of a prominent Democratic holdover. The "two-year" man who had acted as Region VIII's migrant health representative moved on at the termination of his two years.

The structure of the "classical" forces changed somewhat, too. The former Migrant Health Branch chief was "moved upstairs" as rural health advisor to the Community Health Service director; the Region VI migrant health representative retired, the Region IV was reorganized so that the migrant health representative became only one voice among several matters of migrant health.

A headquarters reorganization established a Migrant Health Branch again, and staffed it with many who had been associated with the "classical" period. The leadership was different, however, and the tone of administration distinctly affected by the events of the preceding year. The new leader himself, Billy Sandlin, was a man of about forty, a veteran of the venereal disease program from the Southeast. More ambitious and capable than other venereal disease workers, he had just finished obtaining a Master of Public Health degree, and was somewhat familiar with some modern medical care service concepts. During the MHP controversies, his nature as a conciliator had led him to accept many of the concepts being put forth by the "change-agents," while at the same time maintaining close contacts with the regional offices which were resisting. Although a diffident innovator, he took pride in his ability to "smooth things over" among contending forces and to reduce conflict.

The specific steps this official could take with his branch were clearly circumscribed by what forces came to bear on him from outside. He would respond to his three immediate bosses, the new division director, the CHS director, and the HSMHA administrator. These three officials wanted the program kept quiet. The MHP is a low salience program that few of these officials could see themselves benefiting from. Their business was health, not migrants, and the "action" in health was clearly elsewhere. Furthermore, serving a minority group at this time was not an overly popular enterprise in Washington.

Two sources could give the new Migrant Health Branch chief problems that he would have to handle. First, the new grants were causing controversy in the local areas of award, not inherently of major proportions, as detailed in the next chapter. On the other hand, there remained enough punch left in the "change-agents" so any pronounced retreat would likewise cause problems.

Despite the decimation of their ranks, the "change-agents" retained some influence. A crucial position was manned by the former Alviso Neighborhood Health Center director. He became director of the Migrant Project Group, which was placed in the Office of the Assistant Secretary for Planning and Evaluation in HEW, and was charged with the task of surveying the large range of HEW programs with an eye to improving the share of the migrant in these programs. More informally, this official was able to exercise a good deal of influence even up to the level of the secretary, on occasion, and with the Senate, and was involved in a multitude of actions that helped to keep the MHP in a balancing act. He left this job in the summer of 1971. Another source of continual influence was the "two-year" physician who remained in the MHP, and was somewhat reinforced by a new "two-year" non-physician. The San Francisco regional office was a very powerful advocate of continued change, and could exercise a great deal of direct power by virtue of its direct ties to projects and a large percentage of MHP funds. Its voice in policy discussions within the MHP also carried weight. By the summer of 1971, however, that region had lost several of its young, dynamic personnel.

The new Migrant Health Branch chief, then, was propelled by the MHP history we have outlined, had as an objective to keep the program non-controversial, and found himself in a balancing act between traditional and change forces, although the influence of the latter was clearly diminishing. Luckily for him, little new money was slated to come to the MHP, so he could concentrate on simply defending and manipulating what had already been done, with an eye to minimizing controversy.

Decentralization also had a decided influence. Whereas before it would have been the responsibility of headquarters to set policy *and* carry out that policy, now it had responsibility only for the former. It proved rather easy for headquarters to affirm the previously adopted policy of concentrating resources in large projects, knowing that little money would soon be forthcoming, and knowing that the regional offices by and large could be trusted to administer projects in their old accustomed way, and if they didn't, they would run the risk of blame. Important issues such as sponsorship could well be left to the regions. Thus, the "change-agents" couldn't complain, because many of their prime policies were being endorsed. The conservative regions couldn't complain, because they knew they would have ultimate control over the funds. The San Francisco regional office remained an exception, but their effectiveness tended to diminish with their personnel loss. Finally, the overall lack of funds would ensure that no embarrassments would crop up in new projects.

Along with the directive to decentralize the MHP had come a directive to disband the MHP Project Review Committee, a bulwark of the "classical" forces. It is not clear how the contending forces interacted, but the upshot was an evasion of the order, and reestablishment of the same committee under another name. That this occurred is indicative of the staying power of the "classical" forces.

Headquarters under the new leadership did institute some methodological improvements. Statistics began to be compiled in the central office. Policy planning began to be effected in a relatively overt and concrete manner. The issue of official program guidelines was pursued. Still, these efforts were a far cry from the active support and nurturing of the new projects that might have been attempted. Not one contract, for example, was let for the purpose of consulting with the governing boards of the new projects and advising them as to their functions. No attempts were made to help the new projects with record-keeping methods, scheduling procedures, etc., when experience elsewhere had shown such consultation to be quite valuable to such projects. Neutrality to all projects and concentration of "objective" activities was much the safer course.

This return to "normalcy" brought the federal administrators once again to general administration instead of positive programming. The persons involved were those suited to such a task. This small and insignificant program would not try to change the past, but would try to keep everything rather quiet, with no commotion.

In summary, a marked regrouping of the MHP administration took place after the new projects were established. The "change-agents" lost some key people, general supporters of MHP change in HSMHA were replaced by general opponents, the "classical" faction saw some attrition of power as well, and a Migrant Health Branch was established again, with a new chief of a conciliary outlook. The momentum of change in the MHP affected this new branch, but general balancing requirements were set up by HSMHA influences to keep the MHP quiet and non-controversial, by the threat of disquiet from local areas that had new MHP projects, and residual pressure from "change-agent" sources. Decentralization enabled the Migrant Health Branch to continue the formulation of relatively progressive policies, thus placating the "change-agent" faction, while the responsibility for carrying out the policies fell to the largely conservative regions, thus placating HSMHA and the local area power structures. Lack of increased appropriations also made many of the issues moot. The fact that an HEW order to the effect that the Migrant Health Project Review Committee should be disbanded was evaded points to the continuing influence of the "classical" forces. In general, by 1971 controversy had abated, many of the changes were adopted, and "normalcy" at a new equilibrium point prevailed in the MHP.

IV ORGANIZATIONAL IMPLICATIONS FOR THE FUTURE MHP

A. Personnel and Organizational Conclusions

In the area of personnel, it is theoretically expected (or perhaps defined) and empirically found in the MHP that "conservers" act in a way to minimize the risk of obvious failure even if their actions preclude the chance of significant successes; that they seek to deal with other professional agencies without intruders; and they tend to want to deal with routine matters of administration. "Non-conservers" on the other hand tend to go for a big payoff, are ready to deal outside of traditional professional channels, and are often happy to deal with non-routine, creativity-demanding matters of administration.

Personnel with little understanding of primary medical care organization will not be able by themselves to plan, program, and evaluate projects delivering primary care. They will have to use their own faulty judgment or rely on the advice of others, often by delegating authority to other institutions to operate projects. Personnel who do understand the issues and details of primary medical care administration will be likely to include that as a main component of all planning, will do planning, programming, and evaluation on their own, and will be less likely to rely on the advice of other institutions. Their ties to other medical institutions will still tend to be strong, however, for they often use such institutions as personal reference groups instead of the PHS.

Finally, personnel who have non-migrant backgrounds or backgrounds uninformed by work with poverty groups, will be less likely to deal with consumer groups at any level, less likely to keep the migrants' general situation and best interests in mind, and more likely to favor their own preconceptions rather than the migrants', than personnel who have had a migrant-involved background.

Organizationally, the MHP has always been a low priority item in eyes of HSMHA, and could be safely predicted always to remain so. HSMHA must have a great many other pots on the fire, given the wide involvement of the federal government in the nation's health services, and the MHP covers only a million (or three million including seasonal farm workers) poor, unorganized persons. HSMHA, then, will usually want the MHP to be kept relatively quiet. Very little political "flak" will be worth the effort from HSMHA's point of view. And if the MHP were suddenly to become a large one with a greater priority, a permanent organization like HSMHA would still exert "conserver" influences, fearing the effect of failure on its image and future growth, and would minimize the amount of innovation and political resistance—and hence risk in HSMHA's eyes—thus generated.

HSMHA can still be regarded as essentially a professional type of bureaucracy, even if the professional connections of yesterday—the state and local health departments—have been broken in many areas. It can be expected that other professional institutions will come to be relied on for support. The medical schools and large hospital complexes would be prime candidates at this point. HSMHA would therefore tend to have the MHP projects, if they were to change sponsorship, link up with the large medical institutions, thus solidifying HSMHA's support.

B. Applications to Regional Health Centers

The most promising alternative emerging from Chapter 3 was the regional center idea. As that chapter pointed out, many regional centers (although lacking firm environmental components) were established in 1970. A prime requirement for this movement was an active federal presence; a passive federal presence led to takeover of the program by outside institutions promoting their own goals. An active federal presence presupposes personnel knowledgeable about both medical care and migrants, to avoid relying on other self-interested institutions for program guidance, to avoid identifying more with the medical care professional community than with the migrants, and to avoid unskillful program design with the best of motives.

The new projects of 1970 came about by coincidence. Personnel with unusual qualifications and unusual motivations were concerned with the MHP by accident—the former Alviso director was in HSMHA transiently as the organization was in chaotic change; the former OEO official was assigned to the MHP because 314(e) funded neighborhood health centers were in a stagnant condition; the "two-year" physicians were of good quality because they were chosen by the professional medical care experts who shortly thereafter left the PHS; the San Francisco regional office personnel were capable and motivated because of the organizational change, and assigned to the MHP because 314(e) was stagnating. Furthermore, this crew found itself with new money to spend by the accident of administration and congressional policies. If the usual "conserver" officials had been running the MHP, or if new money had not been forthcoming, there would have been no new projects.

If change to a regional health center based program strategy is to be recommended, an administrative strategy to effect that change by intent instead of accident must be developed. Personnel with the proper characteristics and knowledge for innovation must be attracted, and the organization must permit and encourage them to pursue change. These two elements are interdependent, for only if the organization wants change will change-oriented personnel be attracted. There is a shortage of such persons; only a situation particularly ripe for their talents and needs will attract them. The relatively senior officials are the keys to change. Their presence was essential in 1970; while quite competent and properly motivated, the "two-year" men had insufficient experience to effect change by themselves. Furthermore, "two-year" physicians can be attracted to the PHS as a draft alternative as long as that is a relevant consideration; obtaining the proper "two-year" men is a question of explicit selection by officials already in the program.

The organization must offer a job to be done—there must be money committed to be utilized in a way attractive to these persons. It is most likely that such persons can be best attracted, and can function best, when there is a rather large job to be done, and when several—probably at least half a dozen—can be hired to work at the same time. "Non-conservers" are more attracted to big jobs than little jobs, and most want to be in a like-minded atmosphere, which can only be created by employing several at a time. The organization setting into which they are recruited must also be such that they are assured their efforts will be welcomed and valued by the organization and noticed by their own reference groups. There must be no "conserver" restraints, no high priority programs involving the same field, and no organizational temptation to use the MHP to pay off other organizations. In 1969–1970, the former OEO official and the former Alviso director would not have joined the effort without potential support from above, nor if 314(e) had blossomed significantly.

An organizational setting geared for an innovational job would thus be a prerequisite for attracting the proper type of personnel as well as for getting the job done. Innovational organizational settings, however, are hardly commonplace. Only three possible solutions are mentioned here.

A traditional solution to the problem of the overlooked program is to take it out of the main line of authority and form a unit reporting directly to a high official. New programs of high priority are often treated this way to get them off on the right foot—as a matter of fact, 314(e), the program that contributed so nicely (if inadvertently) to changing the MHP, was begun in just that way. Such a placement ameliorates the "conserver" influence of personnel and organization, lightens the load of competing priorities of other programs, fosters visibility, and can signify a desire for bold action.

Another solution is placement of the program in an organization specifically geared for innovation. In the federal bureaucracy OEO was briefly looked upon as such a creature. Now, however, no such solution seems possible.

Finally, under certain circumstances continuation of the MHP where it now rests would be a feasible option. Change having come once to the MHP, it now rests at a new equilibrium point, with regulations supporting comprehensive, community-based centers, with the influence of the states greatly diminished, and with personnel in several regional offices favorable to such centers. Further innovation could come if the atmosphere of the surrounding organization were progressive but many of the programs were blocked by scarce funds (as was the case in 1970), and if external pressure were applied by migrant advocate groups and the Congress. If the organization cannot fry big fish, little ones such as the MHP will have to do. If the MHP received a large boost in funds while these organizational conditions obtained, progressive programming might be possible.

All three of these possibilities tacitly assume two phases for the MHP, the phase of innovation and the phase of continuation support and management. It is assumed that the different tasks of each phase require different personnel and different organizational settings. If the skills and motivations of "conserver" personnel are unsuited for innovation and aggressive programming, so are the skills and motivations of "non-conservers" unsuited for the painstaking attention to detail and fiscal adequacy that federal administrators traditionally pay. The implication for legislation is clear: instead of the usual pattern of incremental increases in funding each year and the model of steady growth, it makes more sense—in a small program such as this—to structure pulsatile growth with a large increase of funds one year (with specially recruited personnel and a special organizational arrangement, both made possible by the large amount of new money at hand) followed by only cost-of-living increases for a few years.

All three possibilities involve conscious organizational change as the mission changes. Besides abetting the obvious change in function, organizational change makes an important psychological contribution. A prime component of the "conserver" influence is concern for organizational stability. Programs get compromised when the administering organization calculates the effect of program actions on itself rather than on the recipient group. The knowledge of certain organizational death, or at least mutilation, removes that concern.

What the three possibilities do not take cognizance of, is the need for administrators to be responsive to the migrants, and not just to their own reference group. For many programs responsiveness is ensured by direct contact with the beneficiary group, with the latter having the power to go to the Congress or higher administration officials for leverage. The next chapter will explore to what extent the migrants could expect cooperation and sympathy from the Congress. In any case, however, it would be essential for direct communications between the beneficiary group and the administrators to be established.

The MHP Project Review Committee was one model for ensuring that direct contact. A variant that could be devised would consist of three committees, one for each stream, each with some measure of autonomy for conducting its meetings, hiring consultants, and evaluating the MHP as it saw fit. The more autonomy were granted the committee(s), the more involved and knowledgeable the members would become, and the more effective their involvement.

The problem with the MHP Project Review Committee, however, was its composition. If regulations specified that members would be required to represent a bona fide migrant or seasonal agricultural worker group, or to be consumer members of a MHP project, for instance, some true face-to-face contact would be expected.

C. Summary

If regional health centers were to become the policy of the MHP, an active federal presence would be necessary. This activity would be predicated upon "non-conserver" personnel, knowledgeable and experienced with primary medical care organization and the migrant population. Organizationally, the MHP would need an institutional setting that encouraged innovation and resisted the temptation to use the MHP as a payoff to benefit other programs and organizations.

To attract such personnel, there would have to be an attractive job to be done, signified by financial and organizational commitment; a rather large task force type of operation would be appropriate. A new organization reporting to a high official could be established, or under certain conditions partially replicating those in 1970, the MHP could stay where it is. In any case, it is important to recognize that there are two distinct phases for the MHP, the phase of innovation and the phase of support and management. Both different personnel and different organizational forms are necessary for these two distinct phases; therefore, legislation for pulsatile growth rather than incremental growth is indicated. An advisory group to the MHP, to be composed of migrants and direct migrant representatives, and to have some significant autonomy, would also be required.

V SUMMARY OF CHAPTER 4

I. The MHP and its Milieu, 1962–1969

The MHP came into existence just before the federal government became involved in large medical care service programs, and just before the PHS stopped placing firm reliance on state health departments. The PHS was a traditional "conserver" and professional agency with two sources of "non-conserver" personnel: medical care administration experts interested in personal health service programs, and "two-year" PHS officers. The MHP assumed a place of low salience in the medical care world. Placed deep in the PHS bureaucracy, it persisted in traditional practices of small size grants to traditional health department recipients, all administered by "conserver" federal officials, until 1969. The state health departments rendered organizational support in return for MHP respect for traditional state prerogatives. County health departments, partly because of organizational constraints, kept their projects modest and "low profile," and did not become effective purveyors of primary care. The Migrant Health Project Review Committee performed mainly an organizational support role.

II. Migrant Health Program Changes, 1969–1970

A reorganization in 1969 led to the MHP being administered, in the context of very progressive primary medical care programs, by the two kinds of "non-conservers" in the PHS, mainly in headquarters, but also in some regional offices. By coincidence, $6.8 million was allocated on short notice to the MHP in FY 1970, and half of it was programmed in efforts similar to the regional centers idea. It was found that new style projects could be programmed quickly and well, that it was advantageous to deal with groups which did not have well established but wrong ideas of the type and organization of services to be offered, and that recruitment of manpower proved no immediate obstacle. Where both central and regional federal officials were strong, strong project proposals resulted; where both were weak, so were the projects; where they were mixed, the results were variable. Significant migrant input to projects was more likely in the home-base areas.

III. MHP Regrouping, 1970–1971

After establishment of the new projects, personnel adjustments weakened the "change-agents" and a new Migrant Health Branch was set up with a generally conciliatory chief. The mission set for the branch by HSMHA was to keep the MHP quiet. Efforts in central headquarters to adopt some elements of the progressive policies of the year before placated residual "change-agent" interest, while regional office control of programming ensured placation of HSMHA and local area power structures in most instances. By 1971 the MHP had achieved a new point of equilibrium, accepting many new precepts but hesitating to practice them.

IV. Organizational Implications for the Future MHP

If regional health centers were to become the policy of the MHP, an active federal presence would be necessary to initiate them. "Non-conserver" personnel, knowledgeable about both medical care organization and migrants, would have to be placed in an institutional setting encouraging innovation, and resisting the temptation to use the MHP as a payoff to benefit other programs and organizations. To attract such personnel there would have to be an obvious job to be done, signified by financial and organizational commitment; a rather large task force type operation would be appropriate.

A new organization reporting to a high official could be established, or under certain conditions partially replicating those in 1970, the MHP could stay where it is. Both solutions must recognize that there are two distinct phases for the MHP, the phase of innovation and the phase of support and management. Both different personnel and different organizational forms are necessary for these two distinct phases; therefore, legislation for pulsatile growth rather than incremental growth is indicated. An advisory group to the MHP, to be composed of migrants and direct migrant representatives, and to have some significant autonomy, would also be required.

Chapter Five

The Politics of Migrant Health

Considering the politics of the MHP makes apparent the interconnection of migrant health with other policy fields. Even if the MHP appears to be a small ship buffeted about by the winds and seas of other more important and powerful programs and interests, it is always possible to take advantage of these forces to reach a friendly port. Discovery of that process is the goal of the analysis here.

This chapter shall first place the issue of migrant health in the arena of the congressional committee system, then describe the political forces that affect the MHP. Of the several policy spheres that could conceivably affect the health of migrants, it appears that the most weighty influence will be carried by events in the health sphere. The probabilities in health policy changes shall therefore be reviewed, their effect on migrant health analyzed, and the most appropriate disposition of the MHP assessed in light of these probable development.

Finally, an attempt will be made to utilize this chapter's analysis to devise strategies for gaining adoption of the policy changes suggested by previous chapters, and to assess the feasibility of such changes getting made.

I CONGRESSIONAL STRUCTURE AND THE MHP

A conceptual (as opposed to practical) case could be made for placing the issue of migrant health in at least four different specialty areas in the Congress. (All the structural dilemmas listed here apply as well to the administrative branch as to the legislative.) Since the migrant workers are by definition agricultural workers, the committees on agriculture could lay claim to the issue. On the other hand, since migrants are also by definition a part of the labor force, a case could be made for the committees that deal with labor. Since migrants are poor, the committees dealing with problems of poverty could be viewed as appropriate.

Since the issue is the health of migrants, one could say that the committees dealing with health should have jurisdiction. Furthermore, one could argue as to whether all the problems of the migrant should be dealt with in one committee, or the various aspects should be divided up among the various categorical committees.

These are not empty questions. Quite to the contrary, the placement of the issue decides the context in which it is seen, and thus its ultimate disposition. For instance, if the problems of migrants were to be considered in the agricultural committees, they would be seen in the context of farm problems in general, and would compete for attention and money with the farm interests. Although the problems considered would probably be those concerning contributions of the migrants to production, nonetheless, one would be inevitably led to consider a subsidy to migrants in the same light as a subsidy to farmers—that is, as a contribution to the welfare of agriculture—specifically, how much would subsidy of the working force benefit the industry, as opposed to subsidy of other parts of the industry? By way of contrast, if the issue were addressed in the poverty committee, money devoted to migrants would be seen as part of the spectrum of aid delivered to the poor, and their contributions to the economy ignored.

In addition to the contextual variation the different committees would provide, there would also be marked differences in the preconceptions of the committee members. As a rule, for instance, Agriculture Committee members are conservatives concerned with the welfare of farmers, whereas Labor and Public Welfare Committee members are liberals inclined to deal rather generously with those whom they view as abused. On the other hand, the MHP might well appear more congenial to the American consciousness if viewed as an agricultural subsidy than as a poverty subsidy. Other committee placements with different connotations can also be imagined. There are so many variables here, including organizational influences in the Congress, idiosyncrasies of specific members, etc., that serious speculation on the effects of different possible placements for the MHP would have to be based on deeper analysis than that presented here. Such a detailed analysis would probably have little immediate relevance, however, since change of congressional committee jurisdiction does not seem to be a current possibility. Nevertheless, raising the issue of jurisdiction illuminates the arbitrary nature of the current context in which the MHP is viewed. Practically, if one realizes this fact he can gain tactical advantage at times by broadening the scope of discussion to include those factors neglected because of committee placement.

Whether all problems of migrants are considered together, or whether they are considered piecemeal by the categorical committees, clearly bears on the shape of programs to be produced. It is unlikely, for instance, that unified consideration of the problem would produce three separate programs for migrants on "antipoverty," education, and health, and that each of the three programs would allot money for health separately and independently, as is now the case. Likewise, it would be unlikely that an independent and unified migrant committee would produce a health plan fully in step with the rural health plans for the nation (not that categorical consideration necessarily leads to coordination within the category).

The Senate has been better able to solve these organizational dilemmas than the House or the Executive Branch because its members are less specialized. The Committee on Labor and Public Welfare deals with labor questions, health questions (although the Finance Committee has excluded financing jurisdiction over Medicare, Medicaid, and National Health Insurance), and poverty questions, so placing the migrants there kills several birds with one stone. Furthermore, for over ten years the committee has had a Subcommittee on Migratory Labor. Although the subcommittee has the jurisdiction to investigate virtually anything connected with migrants, it has no direct legislative functions; all bills must be considered by the standing legislative subcommittees of the appropriate Senate committee. The MHP is under the jurisdiction of the Health Subcommittee, which takes advice from the Subcommittee on Migratory Labor. The subcommittee does provide, however, an institutional setting for taking a unified overall view of the migrants, where inconsistencies of various programs from the migrants' point of view can be eliminated. Moreover, the subcommittee can act as a lobbying group in itself, constantly reminding other subcommittees and committees of the migrants' existence and arranging for any needed analysis or testimony. The other subcommittees of the parent committee should be particularly susceptible to such influence. The existence of the subcommittee increases the effective salience of the migrant issue.

The Appropriations Committee reflects in its organization the divisions of the substantive committees. The same organizational dilemmas bear on it as on the substantive committees. The MHP is viewed in the Appropriations Committee essentially as a health program for a poor group, and is considered annually along with the entire Health, Education and Welfare package.

In the House of Representatives the MHP is placed along with health legislation (except financing programs such as Medicare, Medicaid, and NHI) in the Subcommittee on Public Health and the Environment of the Interstate and Foreign Commerce Committee. Because of the degree of specialization of the House, not so many relevant fields are unified in this committee as in the Senate's committee; education, agriculture, labor questions, and so on, are all considered elsewhere. In February 1971 a Subcommittee on Agricultural Labor was established in the House Committee on Education and Labor. It has legislative jurisdiction over any bills within the parent committee's jurisdiction that concern primarily farm workers—that is, labor and education issues. The subcommittee seeks to be active in keeping the migrant in mind in current legislation, adding appropriate amendments, as well as monitoring the relevant executive agencies, and initiating its own legislation. For consideration of migrant health, personal contacts exist between the chairmen of the two subcommittees and members. A measure of coordination such as is found in the Senate should be thereby achieved, and the migrants now have an institutionalized "internal lobbyist."

The House Appropriations Committee considers the MHP along with the HEW budget, generally in the context of health programs for the poor, much as in the Senate.

In summary, the MHP finds itself mainly in the health policy area in the Congress, just as it does in the executive. Specific subcommittees exist in both House and Senate to act as unifying overseer of migrant-related legislation. and more importantly as internal lobbying units.

II THE POLITICAL FORCES IN MIGRANT HEALTH

The major forces active in the field of the MHP can best be described by taking an historical view, first describing the political origin of the MHP, then describing the changes in the forces that have occurred since the MHP's initiation. Finally, the dynamics that the forces engage indicated by describing the political reaction to the 1970 reforms.

A. The Original Major Forces in the MHP

1. The Elements. After the demise of the Agricultural Workers Health and Medical Association after World War II, the issue of migrant health was kept active through the 1950s by a few voluntary and religious groups (the Migrant Ministry, National Consumers League), a few health organizations (APHA) and health officers in migrant impact counties (Fresno, California, and Palm Beach, Florida), the Council of State Governments and the Western Governors' Conference, and particularly a governmental official later to become Chief of the Migrant Health Branch for a short time (Helen Johnston). In 1946 the Federal Interagency Committee on Migratory Labor, in 1959 the Association of State and Territorial Health Officers, and in 1960 the President's Committee on Migratory Labor all called for a migrant health program. In 1960 a national TV network show by Edward R. Murrow, called "Harvest of Shame," made a strong impression on public opinion about the unsatisfactory conditions of the lives of migrants. Miss Johnston relates that shortly thereafter, at a meeting of many of these public-spirited persons and groups, Senator Harrison Williams of New Jersey, the first chairman of the Subcommittee on Migratory Labor and apparently influenced by the New Jersey Consumers League, was urged to introduce and support a bill to contribute to the health of migrants. The first version of the Migrant Health Bill was then produced by collaboration of the public-spirited group with one of the Senator's aides. Representative Paul Rogers, advised by his home county health officer, Dr. C.L. Brumback, originated the MHP with similar support in the House.

Through the hearings and committee report that led to the eventual adoption of the bill, efforts were made, as of course they always are, to shape and explain the bill in a way that would elicit the maximum possible support. An examination of the committee report and an interpretation of the bill itself can therefore reveal much about the original political environment.

The Senate and House reports accompanying the original bill in 1961 stress three groups that would stand to benefit from the legislation. First stood the migrant himself, whose poor health and problems in obtaining medical care were mentioned. It was also stressed in this report, however, that several segments of the local communities through which migrants pass would also obtain benefit from the legislation. "Attempts to meet these health needs can become a great burden (both on physical facilities and on the financial resources) on the taxpayers, doctors, and hospitals in these local communities." [1] So local community health providers could expect to benefit.

Health protection of the migrant was also declared to be in the interest of the general public, as in the case of infectious diseases: "A recent diphtheria outbreak among permanent residents in a Texas community was traced to migrant workers." [2]

Finally, the employers of migrants, would be benefited, the report claimed: "Quite apart from humanitarian reasons, these needs should be met in order to assure a continuing supply of efficient and skilled migrant agricultural workers on whom large segments of our nation's agriculture have come to depend." [3]

Widening the constituency is a familiar ploy in shaping legislation; it does however have a cost. Because the interests of the migrants and the other groups with a stake in the legislation will not always coincide, there is bound to be some competition for the allocation of funds. An example of competition would be, for instance, the choice between an extensive immunization campaign that would benefit migrants somewhat and surrounding communities somewhat, or intensive efforts to improve the migrants' nutrition, which would be of more benefit to the migrant (few migrants get diphtheria, many more are malnourished) but of decidedly less to the surrounding community. Another would be the choice between awarding a grant to the county health department, which would be able in some instances to use migrant health resources for more general community purposes, or awarding the grant to an indigenous migrant group, which would not be so inclined. Still another example is the choice of which type of health aide to employ, a charitably inclined local resident, a local college girl interested in nursing, or a migrant. Since the report included non-migrant groups as potential program beneficiaries, it gave official notice to such groups that they have a claim on the funds. Yet, such coalitions are sometimes necessary in trying to pass legislation to benefit a politically weak group.

Besides this overt coalition of interests, we can infer the existence of many other interests. The Association of State and Territorial Health Officers, for instance, which called for a program supporting migrant health in 1959, genuinely wanted the state of health of the migrant improved. They also expected that many of the programs would be run through their members. They regarded such programs as part of their jobs, and were used to working with federal government funds. The payoff for these men would be at least increased staff, increased budget, increased authority, increased power. Their ideological burden, as was discussed elsewhere, inclined them mostly to the status quo, with personal health care kept primarily in the private sector, and with public care offered in "poverty clinics." Resistance to consumer input was also part of their burden.

The same was also true of local health officers. The health officers of the seminal programs in Palm Beach and Fresno counties certainly expected support for their programs, and their favorable testimony was predicated in part on that expectation. Were local health departments not to be frequent recipients of migrant health grants, the support of the state and local health departments for the MHP would cease. The local departments had increased staff and budget to look forward to as much or more than the states.

The persuasions of the local health departments generally match those of the state health departments. In addition, the local health departments must operate within the framework of a local political structure that in rural communities is usually firmly in the hands of the relatively wealthy, including the growers and the private physicians. It has been noted previously that a health department employed ultimately by the county commissioners would find it politically impossible to cite and pursue environmental deficiencies perpetuated by these same commissioners or their allies, especially when the beneficiaries of improvement would be transients with no sanctions to offer. Likewise, since the health department is "the other side of the coin" of the private medical system, no systems of care offering competition or even merely favorable comparison with the services of private medicine are likely to be offered.

In addition, as part of the local political system and "establishment," the health department must be responsive to employment and other considerations dictated by that orientation.

The church groups and other voluntary groups who supported the program also had expectations to be fulfilled. Many expected to be continuing active contributors to the cause, in various ways. They expected to participate in national decision-making, as on an advisory committee. They expected to participate at local levels, possibly with programs of their own. The motivations are familiar; a genuine desire to help the migrant, increased personal and organizational power, and in this case the personal need to participate in humanitarian causes.

The nature of these groups is rather well known. Politically unideological and not inclined directly to challenge dominant forces, they are most inclined to "do good" by consensus. Even though they do not share the objective position of the local health departments, psychologically they stand side by side with them.

The American Public Health Association represented yet another constituency with professional prestige that would lend support to the program, but which had certain objectives that were not exactly coincident with those of the migrant. Serving to some extent as the spokesman of liberal health care theoreticians, researchers, and educators, the APHA was anxious to see the federal government involve itself in providing medical care for civilian Americans, anxious to see experiments in medical care provision take place, and anxious that certainly nothing should happen in the MHP that would jeopardize an expansion of federal efforts to other medical care efforts. The more the federal government involved itself in medical care, the more influence the APHA and its members stood to gain.

Although many elements of the APHA were at this time challenging the dominance of private medicine, only very few were challenging the roles of state and local health departments. In fact, quite the opposite was the case; a great deal of the membership of the APHA was made up of representatives from these agencies, and the rest of the APHA supported them. While the ideological burden of the APHA could be said to vary from those of local and state health departments, in terms of practical support the APHA backed the other agencies.

The final major group lobbying for the MHP was the federal officials who expected to administer it. As with virtually all officials, consideration was placed on security of office. Ability to direct the program to the benefit of potential supporters was therefore one prerequisite, and sufficient latitude to make such direction voluntary on the federal official's part was another, i.e., if it were involuntary to direct a program to a certain group, that group would not be beholden to the director for that act. Furthermore, it was beneficial to the official to have the field of migrant health recognized as a specialty in and of itself, in which the official was recognized to have a certain expertise. The future MHP administrators certainly expected the first condition to be fulfilled by a permissively worded bill, and would encourage the second condition on their own.

The outlook of these officials and others who came into the MHP after it was established, was very much like those of the other groups we have mentioned. They were committed to working without disturbing any powerful groups, and committed to working within the then traditional governmental arrangements.

There were, then, quite a few groups who expected something for themselves from the MHP, although no contradiction was recognized between their claims on the program and the migrants'. It can also be appreciated that the claims of these groups all fit together pretty well.

2. Results of Influence. Many of the provisions in the law and the subsequent actions of the administrators can be traced to motivations that stem from these influences. The private providers of medical care in the local areas were benefited by the usual design and small size of the projects. The type of medical care provided caused no competition with local practitioners, and often provided a referral service. After several years of program operation, the local hospitals benefited by direct payments in return for care of migrants. The general local community as well as the medical providers were benefited by the existence of any program at all–it reinforced their feeling of lack of responsibility for the migrants. They could now say easily: "They're not our responsibility. They're federal people." The interest the projects manifested in immunizations also served to aid the communities, as the House report promised. Some tax relief was probably obtained, and well-meaning persons in some communities sometimes got subsidies for their efforts to help the migrant. In addition, the program strategy of "friendly persuasion" and working through official souces insured a passive political role for the projects that could not upset local political forces in the least.

Growers in the local areas received benefit from the programs by having any possible responsibility for the health of their workers shifted from their shoulders; there was no political cost for the growers here, either, since no form of community organization around the issue of health that might have later political spinoffs was permitted. "Safe" sponsorship of the projects minimized pressure on sanitation, housing, occupational hazards, etc. The Program's charter calling for family clinics rather than emphasizing enforcement of environmental sanitation was another plus for growers.

Local and state health departments received the lion's share of the grant money, as has been shown. With it, they were able to increase their staffs and their power. The projects established, as already described, threatened no one in the local areas, and conformed to the skills the health departments brought to the job.

The Project Review Committee of the MHP conferred welcome duties, including site visit trips, upon many church-related and freestanding MHP advocates, and gave them a vehicle to use in their desire to help others. Some of the voluntary advocates had organizations that received grants for projects. Virtually all were invited to large, annual meetings with a convention atmosphere. The Review Committee also provided a way for the supporting groups to keep watch over the program, and an institution for the administrators to use for support.

The APHA was rewarded with a bill with a progressive sound to it. Family care centers were a relatively progressive concept, as was granting federal funds directly to the operator instead of always through the state. The fact that the MHP did not in fact do anything very progressive was not upsetting to the APHA, which was happy to see a precedent set without any subsequent turmoil. In addition, the APHA in 1963 awarded a contract to study the MHP program operation, which they were happy to accept. The contract per se was helpful to the organization, just for the infusion of money and appearance of activity, and in addition it gave the APHA a chance to have a say in running the program. The fact that the APHA report's critical comments were largely ignored indicates the greater power of the health departments and other groups. The fact that the APHA did not follow up the report shows probably both the low salience of the program, and the ambivalence of the APHA (with its strong health department representation).

The federal officials received their due as well. They were constantly consulted by Congress and were treated as the experts in the field—more on the basis of their lobbying record than any particular expertise with health or migrant labor. The provisions of the law were written with the clear intention that a great deal of discretion over funds dispersal be exercised by the federal administration—a clear advantage for constituency building, as well as a source of satisfaction in itself. They used this discretion to build further support for themselves by giving many grants to many groups, chiefly health departments. The fact that the necessarily small grants were programmatically inefficient was ignored.

It seems clear in hindsight, then, that many groups had a call on the legislation in addition to the migrants. It requires no further elaboration to be assured that each group enumerated above, as a more or less well-organized and practiced lobbying group, was likely to have a closer link in the decision-making process than the unorganized and voiceless migrants. In their role as migrant advocates, most of these groups would be able to press any claims with uncontroverted assertions of those claims "being in the migrants' interest."

The one well-organized group of agricultural laborers, the National Farm Workers Union, and later the United Farmworkers' Organizing Committee, never played a prominent role in the MHP, even though they were included (by departmental fiat) with one representative on the Review Committee. This reluctance to play a role appears to stem from the priorities and beliefs of that union, to devote itself to organizing primarily, and to rely on its own resources.

The migrants were unable to perform the elementary political function of representing themselves as a lobbying group, just as their elementary voting sanction was ineffective. This very fact of helplessness was the precipitant for having a migrant health program in the first place. If the MHP has been ineffective, as Chapter 2 argues it has, many of the reasons for its ineffectiveness (reliance on health departments, dispersion of funds, inadequate attention to quality care) can be traced to that same underlying problem—lack of effective political representation and power. If the initiators of the MHP sought to compensate for the predations of the migrants' exploiters by passing the bill, they neglected to guard against the predations of the migrants' friends in the lobbying process.

B. Political Developments, 1962–71

Through the years, from the early 1960s to the early 1970s, the forces impinging on the MHP changed in a way reflective of the change of the times. The result is a definitely changed political atmosphere today.

The migrants have made some small gains in representing themselves.

UFW is much stronger, if still not interested in mixing with federal programs. Their basic answer to the MHP is to create a health system of their own. AFL-CIO has won the Chavez union as a member, and gives some support (although often not wholehearted) to them in Congress. Some other organizations of farmworkers have sprung up, the most prominent being Colonias de la Valle in the Lower Rio Grande Valley, Texas, and Organized Migrants in Community Action (OMICA), in Homestead, Florida. The movement for self-organization is similar to that of other underprivileged minorities, although the force is much weaker. Basically locally-oriented groups, Colonias and OMICA can exert some influence in their home counties, but on the national scene they have had quite limited impact.

The decade has also seen the rapid growth of the new, consciously non-paternalistic advocacy groups, both privately and publicly funded. The Colorado Migrant Council gives direct service and employs advocacy techniques. California Rural Legal Assistance, Colorado Rural Legal Assistance, Florida Rural Legal Assistance, and the Migrant Legal Action Program use the force of law to protect migrants, and the latter uses its influence in the legislative and administrative areas.[a] Rallying public opinion through publicity is the major *modus operandi* of the Center for Community Change and the Field Foundation. Although these groups do not represent a great deal of "hard" political clout—votes and/or money—their addition to the field has changed the atmosphere and informational content of the field.

The media have increasingly pointed out migrant problems, high points being an NBC documentary in 1970 emphasizing that conditions had changed little since Edward R. Murrow's program ten years before, and a *New York Times* series of articles in 1971. Appeal to public opinion is, of course, the major objective of such efforts.

As the medical care political situation has changed, so have the positions of those groups mainly concerned with medical care. The APHA is not looking to set the same precedents now as before. They are not concerned about marginal increases in federal financial involvement in medical care, nor in breaking down the federal-state-local government pipeline. Rather, they are interested in experimentation with new organizational arrangements for medical care, using new types of personnel, etc. Many are concerned with experiments in community participation, and with putting special emphasis on poor groups. The influence of the health departments has decreased somewhat.

The AMA has backed away considerably from its adamant stand against federal interference with health and against organized forms of practice. The chairman of the Rural Health Council, also a member of the MHP Review Committee, has put himself on record as favoring the regional approach to rural health, and the utilization of group practice in these areas. They did, however,

[a] The compromise legal services bill signed into law by President Nixon in 1974 abolishes federal support for all back-up centers, including MLAP, as of the end of that year.

pass a resolution in their 1970 convention condemning the MHP's recent innovations.

The politics of the Nixon Administration can hardly be said to be favorable for migrant health, with the emphasis on budget cutting in health and the general turn away from antipoverty programs. On the other hand, Chicanos have been looked upon as a potentially Republican group, and the MHP relatively favorably regarded as a consequence, so long as the MHP efforts remain rather conventional. Much of the relevant maneuvering remains in secrecy at this point, but it seems likely that the explanation for the MHP's receiving good increases in funding during the Nixon years lies in those political perceptions.[b] In general in the health field, the administration has progressed with the field in espousing national health insurance, finally, and the initiation of health maintenance organizations.

Organizationally, HEW has much attenuated ties with state health departments. Its perceptions on health service projects have been drastically refocused by the 1960s experiences. "Radicalism" is defined by the militancy of grant recipients; giving grants to indigenous non-governmental organizations is no longer radical, so long as those groups are not confrontational.

The Congress has changed as well. The Senate Subcommittee on Migratory Labor evolved from the liberal Harrison Williams to a more radically sympathetic Walter Mondale, who pressed for strong consumer participation in migrant health projects. The basic constituency structure has remained unchanged, however, and probably only a Northerner can afford to make anything of the position. In giving up his post for another, Mondale advised Alan Cranston of California not to take the position, since a state like California, even with all its migrants, did not have sufficient constituent attractiveness. That is to say, the forces against the migrant would be so strong on Cranston he would be politically unable to make anything out of the job. Adlai Stevenson III, even though subject to some downstate pressure, made a more apt chairman, as has Gaylord Nelson, the current incumbent. It is indicative of the saliency of the migrant issue, however, that the chairmanship is so often delegated to a junior member, and changes hands so frequently.

The Subcommittee on Health has seen marked change as Edward Kennedy in 1971 replaced the defeated Ralph Yarborough of Texas as chairman, and as the political stakes and visibility of the health issue have continued to rise on their own, and by virtue of the entry of the powerful Kennedy. Kennedy has been aggressive on health, using it to display his liberalism and capacity as a legislator. Unbeatable in Massachusetts, Kennedy has kept his presidential options alive by fostering an image of competence and liberalism. Keeping no enemies on the Left, he tries to extend his positions as far to the middle as possible, and to

[b] Fred Malek, an HEW power during the first Nixon administration, has recently been revealed as having advocated that grants programs be made politically "responsive." It is possible the MHP was one target.

compromise sufficiently to be able to cite accomplishments. He has used the health issue in just this way, staking out Left positions on national health insurance, health maintenance organizations, and other issues, and compromising from these. The definition of "Left" is sometimes shaky, but is generally defined by an issue's adherents, and usually includes more money, more help to the poor, less concern about cost controls, less protection against "bad acting" consumers and more against "bad acting" professionals, and more emphasis on explicitly defining systems of care.

The Kennedy personal and Health Committee staffs are by general reputation rather ideological. They fit together well with Kennedy, since they can stake out the Left positions, with his support, and he can compromise them as necessary. To compromise is his natural tendency anyway, and doing so makes him attractive to his fellow politicians. The health staff with two exceptions is not well liked nor much respected for ability and capacity to relate well personally, by the other staffers on health issues in the House and Senate. They are often criticized for sloppiness in drafting bills, and obtuseness in dealing with technical issues. The Kennedy staffers tend to criticize the others as insufficiently liberal. The MHP legislation is handled in tandem by the Health Committee Staff and Kennedy's staff assistant for Chicano affairs.

Both emotionally and politically, Ted Kennedy inherits a special constituency in the Chicano farmworkers from his brother Bobby, who was closely tied to Cesar Chavez. Yarborough had farmworkers as part of his essential Texas constituency; although they are objectively less important to Kennedy, they are more important symbolically, and he is unhampered by concerns of the growers and the surrounding communities that might have inhibited Yarborough.

Interference with the work of the Health Subcommittee by the parent Labor Committee is small. The MHP does get some special attention, however, since Harrison Williams, the MHP's original sponsor, is now committee chairman. The MHP legislation therefore, receives special attention and support if needed.

Just as the Senate has changed in ways generally favorable to migrants, the House has not been unresponsive. In 1971 the House added a Subcommittee on Agricultural Labor to its Labor and Education Committee. Headed by Northern liberals, it has served to increase the visibility of migrants in the House, but has not ventured much into the field of health.

The real key to the MHP in the House is Representative Paul Rogers, a Democrat representing Palm Beach County and part of Broward County in Florida since being appointed to succeed his father in 1954.[4] Chairman of the Subcommittee on Public Health and the Environment since 1971, his home district serves as home base to about 30,000 migrants. The Palm Beach County Health Department initiated an experimental migrant health project before the MHP was started; and Rogers was the original House sponsor of the MHP legislation in 1962. So, despite the specialization of functions in the House, migrants and health merge in the person of Representative Rogers.

Several options for further ambitions confront a member of the House. For many years it was not clear what Rogers' choice would be. Able and energetic, he served on the Public Works Committee in his early years in the House, promoting water resources and highways in Florida. Later, as a member of the Interstate and Foreign Commerce Committee and its Subcommittee on Health and Public Welfare, he involved himself in health affairs. Only with a chairmanship can a member of the House flourish, however, and despite his sixteen years of seniority by 1970, it was not clear that a chairmanship would be his. He entertained notions of running for the Senate in 1970, but did not. Instead, when the House adopted a rule confirming each member to only one chairmanship, Rogers found the Health chair suddenly open.

Rogers had been the predominant member of that subcommittee for a few years previously acting virtually as chairman, and so had a running start. He devoted himself to being a "health statesman," somewhat in the mode of Representative John E. Fogarty, previous chairman of the House Labor-HEW Appropriations Subcommittee, or Senator Lister Hill, chairman of the Labor Committee in the Senate. On being named chairman he displayed his organizational astuteness by having the subcommittee renamed as the Public Health and Environment Subcommittee, thus gaining jurisdiction in an important extra area.

Most of Rogers' aspirations now seem to lie with the health field. A next step up would be as a high official in a Democratic HEW, or perhaps secretary of a newly created Department of Health (creation of which Representative Rogers supports). It is important to him, then, that he appear knowledgeable and creative to the various components of the health establishment. In the eyes of the Democratic party, the health establishment includes not so much the conservative American Medical Association as the more liberal—although no less self-interested—Association of American Medical Colleges, American Hospital Association, American Public Health Association, Blue Cross and Blue Shield, and many more. Rogers interprets his task as being, first, to merit respect by the establishment for his ability and energy, and second, to be viewed as an ally (or at least not an enemy) by as many of these organizations and persons as possible. In practice, he is quite adept at achieving respect as a health politician-statesman. He knows issues well, especially which groups feel which way about them. He chooses legislation rather progressively, brokers among the various organizations sensitively to achieve consensus, and manages bills well in the House and in negotiations with the Senate and administration. He sees his role politically, rather than academically or intellectually, so he can readily adopt another's proposal as his own, no matter where it comes from.

Rogers' own politics are conservative; he generally opposes OEO-type efforts, but on the local level has characteristically sought to mediate between

Migrant Legal Service representatives and the establishment. Like Lister Hill, however, the general tenor of his politics is not reflected in his attitude towards health legislation—he finds himself comfortably in the middle of the generally "liberal" health establishment on almost all issues. The House is almost always more conservative about expenditures than the Senate; in this way, too, Rogers finds himself in the mainstream.

Like Kennedy, Rogers has a special interest in migrants. Since sponsoring the original legislation, he has been a key figure in its renewal and growth through the years, and has frequently been personally involved in migrant health issues in South Florida, seeking to mediate agreements among local officials, federal officials, local physicians, local hospitals, and the state health department.

Just as he seeks consensus on issues within the health establishment, Rogers seeks consensus within his subcommittee. Several of the members are rather active in health legislation, notably Democrat William Roy of Topeka, Kansas (a physician), and Republican James Hastings of upstate New York. Rogers is responsive and cooperative with these men, and often shares sponsorship in Roy-Rogers bills on the former's initiative. Collectively, they share Rogers' generally pragmatic viewpoint.

The staff of the subcommittee and several of the members work cooperatively, are pragmatic and non-doctrinaire, and reflect the philosophy of their bosses. They are less clique-ish and more conservative than the Kennedy staffers.

Rogers and Kennedy are thus the two congressional kingpins. Both have an interest in Kennedy's appearing to be further to the left. Kennedy needs the Left for his national constituency, and Rogers needs to be to the right of Kennedy for his own local constituency. Both, however, need to appear responsible and reasonable. As Democrats facing a hostile Republican administration, both have a further incentive to cooperate; indeed, their effectiveness depends on a certain degree of cooperation. Finding a common ground against the Nixon administration is fairly easy for most Democrats; for health advocates, it is particularly easy to oppose the cost-cutting approach of the Nixonians. In a crunch, Kennedy would be able to stick with a migrant program attached by Conservatives, because of its positive symbolic power for him. Rogers, on the other hand, would back off, for he needs a consensus in order to bolster his health constituency, and must not be too Leftish for the folks back home.

In summary, the advocacy atmosphere surrounding the migrant has received a strong admixture of young, progressive lawyers, and some groups of migrants are now available to speak for themselves. The basic lack of sanctions to apply to elected representatives (votes or money) still exists, however, and reference must still be had to broad public opinion, and some also to the force of law at the local level.

Health policy has seen major changes, and this has been a direct effect on the migrant health policy area. The APHA has become firmer in its interest in health care experiments, firmer in its support of health programs for the poor, and less strongly committed to health departments. The AMA has softened its opposition to group practice, and has even come to support federal monies in health. HEW, now Republican, is firmly committed to federal involvement in health care financing and organization, no longer deals reflexively with state health departments and has sought to cut costs in health. Chicanos have been a Nixon political target (as potential friends, not enemies); MHP funding has prospered as a result. Congress has also become committed to federal involvement in health care. Kennedy in the Senate and Rogers in the House have emerged as major powers. Both are very conscious of the issue of migrant health, although their major interests lie with the larger health issues. Rogers has aspirations to be a major health statesman, and is committed to the established health forces, although not to any one in particular. Kennedy has a national liberal constituency, and migrants are a pet symbolic issue. Throughout all these changes, the MHP has remained a generally popular and non-offensive program, the more so since the definition of "radical" has undergone change.

C. Political Dynamics—The Case of the 1970 Reforms

A taste of the dynamics of MHP politics can be obtained by briefly considering the political events surrounding the MHP change in strategy of 1970. It will be remembered (see pp. 122–130) that the strategy change was heralded by rather widespread circulation of a new set of guidelines in 1969, and then a very rapid awarding of grants to new types of grantees in the spring of 1970, after a late HEW appropriation by Congress.

The change in strategy was complicated by the personal power struggle within the bureaucracy. The former Migrant Health Branch chief, by this time only a rural health care advisor to the division chief, employed familiar means of seeking to reassert her power. Her old ties to the Senate were called upon, and in answering planted questions at the Migrant Health Hearings in 1969 (her presence was deemed necessary at the hearings, even though she no longer ran the MHP—a sign of her residual power), strongly implied that the MHP was being slighted by the new organizational arrangement. The Health Subcommittee subsequently recommended in their report that the Migrant Health Branch be reestablished.

A second source of influence the former branch chief called upon was some members of the MHP Review Committee, and associated old backers of the MHP. Letters were directed to the Senate and referred thence to HEW for response. They expressed alarm that old MHP policies were to be changed, and alarm that young, inexperienced physicians and others had achieved a position of influence in the MHP.

The former Migrant Health Branch chief also tried to use her influence to concentrate opposition on the new Guidelines. How much of the actual response to the Guidelines was instigated by the former branch chief cannot be assessed, since it was the policy of the Guidelines proponents to circulate them widely and gain adherence by consensus. Many state health departments reacted with some concern, usually with letters to the PHS regional offices, occasionally involving representatives in Congress, but since the Guidelines were never issued officially, reaction could never be taken too far in political channels. The best judgment on the Guidelines reaction would probably be that the "change-agent's" strategy of openness blunted an effective counterattack on that issue by the former branch chief, because the appearance of personal pique could not be avoided, whereas had the Guidelines been kept secret and leaked through this official, the objective situation would have appeared more threatening to the health departments, and they would have lined up behind an old ally more willingly. As it was, they were mostly willing to wait and see.

The most potent force the former branch chief could bring to bear was the regional representatives. They were a major restraining force in policy changes, but acted in a bureaucratic rather than political way. The pressure brought to bear from the outside on the former branch chief's initiative was in fact minimal, and rather easily cushioned by the bureaucracy. The source of her power was mostly bureaucratic.

The real outside power sources were only revealed when it became apparent that the newly appropriated money would be used for new types of projects that would be threatening to several constituencies. The "change-agents" realized that some of the new money would have to be spent to appease some constituencies; their superiors realized this even more. Accordingly, half the funds were allotted to traditional projects run by state health departments, the Palm Beach County Health Department project in Congressman Rogers' home district, and much to the dismay of the "change-agents," a non-descript "communications in the stream" project to be run by a Catholic Sisters organization allied with the former branch chief. The remainder of the money was used for projects of the new type, with grantees of a new type. It was these projects which provoked political responses that can be examined with profit. It should be remembered that the time frame for the project granting process was very short, and thus the opposition often had insufficient time to mobilize. The fact that only one project was actually blocked reflects this specific tactical situation, rather than overall power relationships.

In the local areas hosting new projects, the most active and effective opposition came consistently from physicians and health groups, and sometimes from local governmental units. The major threats the doctors saw were direct competition for patients and new forms of organization in their backyard. In some cases the physicians were joined by allies such as the local pharmacist. They had several avenues through which to carry their protests. They used their professional organizations to assert pressure where possible. The AMA national convention passed a resolution submitted by the California delegation condemning the new MHP policy.

At the county level several medical societies approached their congressman, who proved sympathetic to the physicians in every case. Generally, one could say, the congressman looked to the local medical society as the key unit to indicate what his stand should be. In some cases, the local physicians sought and obtained sympathetic contacts at high levels in HSMHA and HEW. Two particular factors made these levels susceptible to the physicians' influence. The HSMHA administrator felt special sensitivity for reasons mentioned in the preceding chapter—basically, he held a higher priority for other programs for which he would need to stockpile physician support. A Deputy Assistant Secretary for Health and Scientific Affairs with political ambitions felt sensitivity as a representative of the Nixon Administration that would, of course, value physician support. Although these top officials would have trouble in asserting their will completely over a unit (the MHP) several levels below them, no one would doubt that they could do so, sooner or later. Only the speed with which the grants were awarded prevented several of the projects from being vetoed.

Local physicians often treated directly with the Federal Regional Office responsible for the project. Although grant adjustments were sometimes made as a result, in general these were not productive contacts. The physicians were out to kill the projects, not change them, so negotiations would not work. The pressure of the doctors could only be brought to bear on the regional office in a roundabout way through Congress or the higher levels of the bureaucracy (because the regional offices were not yet run by administration people); because such efforts took time to develop, the projects survived. A somewhat unusual tactic was taken in the Imperial Valley, where a group of physicians actually brought suit against HEW for mounting a project in an allegedly inappropriate area. (The suit lost.) Still other actions were taken at the local level in trying to build community opposition, generally without success.

Local health departments and state health departments were understandably major opponents of new type projects on their own turf. They had more difficulty than the private physicians in enlisting support from their professional organization, for the APHA is much more diverse than the AMA. The top leadership, in particular, are not tied to the health departments as an important constituency. The other professional ties of these health departments, to the PHS, were precisely the source of the problem. Now that they were having trouble with these ties, it left them in a quandary as to what to do. Formal letters of protest to HSMHA at various levels were sent, and some inquiries made through congressmen. Since the health departments do not count for much politically, these contacts were much less fruitful than those of the private physicians. Some congressmen looked at the local health department for signals on the new projects, but certainly accorded less weight to these views than those of the medical societies. Their traditional hold on the PHS and HSMHA probably had some general effect in confirming the HSMHA administrator's decision to clamp down on the changes, but the pressures from the Congress and private medicine were more salient.

As an interesting example, in Homestead, Florida, project support was obtained from all local medical components (the medical society, medical school, Health Planning Agency, and county hospital) except the Dade County Health Department, which combined with an already disgruntled Florida State Board of Health to try to intimidate the project. They soon realized, however, that the local forces supporting the project counted for much more than the health departments, and they moved grudgingly to a posture of distant cooperation. Had they been a county medical society, they would probably have been able to extract concessions.

The third significant force that exerted itself at the local level were the local governments themselves. Not involved so often as the first two forces, they did on occasion view a federal grant to an independent body as an OEO-type attempt to set up alternative centers of power. Since the grants were at about the $400,000–$500,000 level, the level of influence gained would be considerable. Their avenues for exercise of influence were not much different from those available to the other groups. A politically significant body such as a county board of supervisors, or a city council, has access to the congressman as well as state government offices. Generally, local governments responded less frequently and less intensively than the medical groups; when they did respond, they added to the establishment forces that stood against the project.

Taken together, all these forces—medical societies, state and local health departments, some local governments, and congressmen—in California apparently had a marked effect on the state governmental policy at a very high level. The Reagan Administration, closely linked with the Nixon Administration, was reported to bring strong pressure to bear on the PHS to force retirement punitively on the ailing older member of the "change-agent" group. If this allegation is true, as the author has reason to believe, this shows graphically how dangerous it was for career members of the PHS to involve themselves in controversial activity. Balancing the outside power to resist change were the centralized bureaucratic "change-agents."

The team of young officials from the HEW Office of the Assistant Secretary for Planning and Evaluation who were assigned to arrange for outside evaluation of the MHP, were soon won over to the "change-agents'" point of view. In early 1970 one of the "change-agents" was transferred from HSMHA to ASPE to head a special project group concerning migrants. This office soon became the HEW center for migrant information. As such, when outside criticism started rolling in, and when the new HSHMA administrator himself agreed with these criticisms, the "change-agents" point of view could be communicated to the Secretary and his surrounding aides.

The young chief counsel to the Senate Subcommittee on Migratory Labor, himself influenced by Washington-based foundations of the "new advocate" sort and supported by Chairman Mondale, was able to write letters (or send letters actually written by the "change-agents") to the HEW administration exerting counter-pressure. Several high HSMHA officials surviving from the previous regime and the California regional office also provided support.

The recurrent theme of young versus old should not be ignored. Not only did the young consider themselves more upwardly mobile, and thus favorable to change, but a real cultural and ideological split from previous, more directive (or "paternalistic") beliefs was probably involved.

Little outside support was forthcoming. The new projects that had a substantial establishment base were able to produce support for their projects (but not the strategy change in general) in the Congress and the regional offices. But projects that were based on consumer groups were able to generate little support, even if they were able to produce large supportive petitions from the community to the congressman or HSMHA officials. In the rural, conservative counties, the congressman knew it was not his constituency talking. Support that would have been effective in other administrations, such as from California Rural Legal Assistance, found little outlet in 1970. The only channel open to the community groups and advocates was to Senator Mondale.

The "change-agents" did not concentrate, as they might have, on producing political support for their changes. They relied rather on quick action, and felt that the outside support they could muster would not be very impressive, and was unnecessary for their limited goals. They feared, further, that too much commotion might bring too much attention and hamper their efforts. Their inexperience and newness to the MHP field might also have been a factor.

They could have orchestrated a write-in campaign to Representative Rogers, Senators Yarborough (chairman of Health Subcommittee and full labor committee) and Mondale, and various HEW and HSMHA officials supporting all the changes, not just the single project the supporters had contact with. Support that was latent could have become manifest. Health departments in Michigan that got big awards could have been mobilized, and perhaps the APHA could have been goaded into support. (In fact, specific use of the prestige of a prominent APHA member and Professor of Medical Care was made by the "change-agents" at several meetings of the MHP Review Committee. The general move toward large projects and consumer participation actually was accepted by the Review Committee, the professor's influence being a crucial ingredient to this unexpected result.) Letter writing campaigns of ordinary citizens in the service areas of the new projects, concentrating on their congressmen and organized by the project grantees, might have been effective. In general, though, most of the support the "change-agents" could be expected to be effective would be from groups other than those they were most intent to help; the projects with marginal value to the program itself had most to offer politically. Furthermore, no thought was given to influencing those not already inclined to a positive point of view. Since the "change-agents" did not actively seek a new, active constituency, it is hard to judge how effective that approach could have been. But most one could have hoped for from most congressmen would have been neutrality or lukewarm support, since the establishment opposition was strong, and had traditional ties to their congressman.

If little outside support was generated, at least the "change-agents" took care to neutralize some groups either by leaving them alone or granting them a little more money. These groups included the whole state of Texas, most of Florida, all the Midwest, Oregon, the Southeast, New York, Michigan, New Jersey, and others. In other words, the great majority of areas were not at all affected by the changes. Since new money, not old money, was dealt with, and since the new money was used in large chunks, only a few areas were upset. California was by far most affected, followed by Washington, Colorado, and South Florida. The possible extent of opposition can be appreciated by considering all the medical societies and health departments who could also have been involved. In addition, some other traditional supporters of the MHP, the voluntary and religious organizations, shared the new money.

The link from a congressman to the executive branch depended very much on the accident of party and congressional status of the individual congressman. Most all were conservatives and inclined to view their constituency and allies as the local medical society, pharmacists, and local officials, and these were opposed to the projects. The party of the congressman made a difference in his access to the executive. The Republican congresswoman from the Yakima Valley in Washington had her objections to that project relayed to HEW by Vice-President Agnew; Republican Congressman Mathias from Tulare-Kern Counties was able to exert firm and unrelenting pressure on the much abused Bakersfield project. The Imperial Valley project was funded while its congressman, John Tunney, was running for senator. While it received no support, the physician opposition had no effective conduit of influence, and chose an unfruitful court challenge instead. In Fresno County the congressman was Bernie Sisk, a maverick Democrat, who was opposed to funding a project that would promote a new center of power in his district. His access to HEW being rather limited, however, he chose to have his aide make personal contact with a "change-agent" in the MHP, and later even made a phone call himself. This sort of intervention, lacking immediately obvious sanctions, proved to be ineffective.

Organizational position was also important for the effectiveness a congressman could enjoy. Clearly, Congressman Rogers' key placement assured his district of a share of additional funds, pretty much on their terms. Organizational placement also insured Senate Majority Leader Mansfield a small grant award to Montana, although the amount involved was so small one cannot attribute too much importance to this gesture on the part of the Denver regional office. Had Senator Mondale wished to be an advocate for any homestate projects, it would have been funded as he wished. The Colorado opposition to the Weld County project might have used Republican Senator Peter Dominick, a conservative member of the Migrant Subcommittee, a good advantage, but to the author's knowledge they didn't. The explanation for this lack might be that the head of the Colorado Health Department was a new member of the MHP Review Committee, and was anxious to protect his position there and did not want to offend the MHP. Perhaps, too, an organ of state government, such as the health department, cannot easily deal with congressional politics.

In practice, with the exception of Representative Rogers' district, no areas of the country were prescribed or proscribed for action by the "change-agents" according to congressional representation. Rather the regional office character and the presence of likely sponsors in a local area were of paramount importance, and the congressional chips were let fall as they might.

It is rather difficult to untangle the next link in the chain of influence, the Office of the Secretary of HEW. On the one hand, the Office of Assistant Secretary for Planning and Evaluation supported the MHP changes. On the other, politically ambitious members of the Office of the Assistant Secretary for Health and Scientific Affairs were eager to be politically responsive to both Republican members of Congress and the interests of the AMA. The HSMHA administrator made opposition representations to the secretary. The secretary himself, who had personal knowledge of the controversy, was doubtless pulled both ways. His interests, however, certainly met those of the HSMHA administrator in wanting the controversy to cool down so as not to impede other, more important matters. The Community Health Service deputy director, who was in active charge of the CHS, felt the same way. Although not subject to political pressures directly himself, he felt them indirectly from the HEW and HSMHA levels. He saw nothing to gain by supporting the MHP changes, and was anxious to promote administrative and political harmony by de-controversializing the MHP. In the context, de-controversializing meant not offending the dominant interest groups.

Probably the main responsibility for de-controversializing the MHP lies at the HSMHA and CHS levels. They responded to political pressure from above, to the HSMHA administrator's preconceptions about desirable power relations in health programs in communities, and to a set of priorities that ranked the MHP low.

If there had been a long lead time on the projects, and if the channels of resistance had had months to operate before grants were awarded, no doubt the easiest method for de-controversialization would have been to block the grant awards. Once awarded, however, the grants were technically difficult to discontinue, and discontinuation would have been embarrassing for the regional offices that had supported the projects, as well as politically embarrassing for the administration. The grants were let to stand, then, although the Kern County project was temporarily suspended on the tenable grounds of the grantees incapacity to fulfill the terms of the grant—although the deeper reason was probably unremitting pressure from Congressman Mathias.

Other steps were taken to de-controversialize the MHP permanently. Although the concept of large grants was accepted, it was made clear to the MHP that establishment grantees should be favored in the future. Headquarters personnel were changed to a more traditional sort in an attempt to assure adherence to the above strictures. A Migrant Health Branch was reestablished to damper possible congressional criticism, to pick up support from the "classical" faction, and to better delimit participation in the MHP administration. Since the MHP administration was largely decentralized to the regional offices in the spring of 1970 subsequent policy in choosing grantees could vary significantly according to the region. As before, only the San Francisco regional office remained equipped and inclined to support new groups. Although they were able subsequently to transfer funds from old projects to the new ones, whether they would be able to do more remained moot, as few new funds became available. With all these steps, plus reassuring statements to the complaining parties, the HEW and HSMHA administrators cooled the crisis down quickly.

In response to the 1970 new projects, then, the most important pressures brought to bear locally against the projects were those of the local physicians; state and local health departments and some local governmental bodies also contributed. The physicians went through their national professional organization, either directly or by implication, and activited the administration directly. The second important pathway of influence was through the local congressman, who was always deferential to the opinions and interests of the local physicians. The congressman's effect on the executive branch varied with his party and organizational placement in the Congress. The most important support for change came from progressive sources, mostly young, within the bureaucracy and Congress, for the most part connected directly with the issue of migrants or migrant health, but not with health in general; it is difficult to tell if outside support in significant amounts could have been supplied, for there was no attempt to do so. For the most part it seemed that project sponsorship, rather than project design, determined the tenor of local response. The conflicting signals converged at the HEW level, which seems not to have given a clear signal to the HSMHA level. The decision to de-controversialize was probably taken at the HSMHA level, but had the tacit consent of the HEW level. The major influences on the HSMHA decision were probably the conservative beliefs of the administrator on proper sponsoring agencies for local projects, a general sensitivity to political criticism, and the low priority of the MHP which militated against going out on a limb for it.

D. Summary

It was apparent from the original reports accompanying the Migrant Health Act that not only migrants, but also local medical care providers, the local community in general, and growers would benefit. The supporters of the legislation would also benefit: state and local health departments, church groups and public spirited citizens, the APHA, and federal officials. The writing of the law and its subsequent administration favored these groups often at the expense of the migrants. The political communications and exchange system operated to include all these groups, but not the migrants, who themselves had no effective lobbying group directly responsible to them. Many program decisions in the MHP's administration that seemed inexplicable from the health administration standpoint are thus explainable from the political viewpoint.

In years following the MHP's establishment, both the general political atmosphere and the specific forces impinging on the MHP changed. Several migrant groups with local roots were organized, and several new migrant advocacy groups came into existence. The APHA increasingly favored medical care experimentation and serving the poor; the AMA softened considerably its opposition to alternative forms of practicing medicine. The general position of health departments vis-à-vis federal programs weakened considerably. Under the Nixon Administration HEW favored the poor less, but viewed Chicanos favorably and supported HMO's under professional auspices. Senator Edward Kennedy became the health and MHP advocate in the Senate, as did Representative Paul Rogers in the House. Although their motives differ, both support the MHP strongly, and both favor reorganization of medical care delivery. Throughout all, the MHP continued to be considered popular and non-offensive.

Brief consideration of the political events surrounding the 1970 MHP innovations reveals some of the dynamics of politics concerning the MHP. Although health departments and local governmental units sometimes opposed the new projects, those most constantly opposed and wielding the most power were the local physicians. Strong objections seemed to correlate best with sponsorship by community groups rather than with type of project design. One route of physician influence was through the national organization, actually or by implication; this route led directly to the federal administration. The other important route of influence was through the local congressman, who was always ready to support the views of the local medical society. The congressman's actual effectiveness depended on his political party and his organizational placement in the Congress. Support for the new projects came mainly internally from young liberals in the federal government. While the HEW level thus got conflicting signals, it gave tacit support for the HSMHA level decision to de-controversialize—that is, "de-aggressivize"—the MHP. The major influences at the HSMHA level were probably the conservative beliefs of the HSMHA administrator on local project sponsorship, a general unwillingness to incur political opposition, and a specific desire to stockpile medical-political goodwill for major programs even if at the expense of low-priority items like the MHP.

III HEALTH CARE POLICY TRENDS

The MHP is for the most part a subset of the health policy area. The trends in health policy therefore determine what policy options and tactical options exist for the MHP. The object of this section is to discuss the current state of health policy. The next section will delineate the implications for the MHP.

The most notable recent change in the health policy area is in the prominence of the problem. Although medical care specialists tried for many years to impress governmental authorities and the public that medical care was being delivered to Americans at standards, cost, and extent far from optimal, only recently has this problem been widely recognized. Although deficiencies in medical care for some groups was appreciated for some time, now the problem is seen to affect all classes.

The most prominent issue is by all accounts *cost*. The cost problem can be seen from two standpoints: the individual's and society's. Individuals are finding medical care often prohibitively expensive, both for insurance premiums, for out-of-pocket expenses for routine and simple illness care (with or without insurance), and for catastrophic episodes of care. From the society's point of view, increasing portions of the GNP (now about 7.4 percent) are being devoted to medical care, both because of high inflation in that sector, because of increases in technology and productivity possibility, and because of an aging population. Increasing cost is the problem most palpable to individuals and politicians alike.

Another very prominent issue is that of *equality*. While one part of the American Ethic calls for an equal chance for everyone and humanitarianism, another calls for free market rule of dollars and economic power. While in one sense it is iniquitous for different persons to have unequal access to medical care, in another sense it is iniquitous for one person to pay for another's care. Under the Johnson Administration an attempt was made to tip the scales in favor of equality of access to care for all, by declaring health care to be a "right of all Americans." Although few public officials dare deny this proclamation, many try to tip the scales the other way by concentrating more on financial equity. In any event, the issue is clearly an extremely hot one that few dare face head-on. Advocates of financial equity speak of doing well for the poor in *their* separate program, and advocates of equality speak of providing more care to needy areas and building up resources, but avoid implications of less or worse, or at least not better, care for the currently favored classes. No one denies, however, that medical care is distributed very unevenly throughout American society, basically according to wealth but also according to other factors such as location and race. And no one denies that the statistics of health are better in the favored communities.

A third area of import can be called *appropriateness of service.* To obtain acceptable primary care service has become more and more difficult for families of all classes—this problem is usually called the "disappearance of the GP." The type of care commonly dispensed has often been attacked as inappropriately favoring treatment over prevention, and surgical over medical therapy. Lack of coordination and continuity of care among the many specialists often consulted has produced similar disquiet. Questions about the competence of many physicians, either because they are unqualified for some of the services they seek to provide, and/or because there is no effective review of a physician's professional actions, have also arisen more and more—often by way of malpractice suits.

The upshot of these problems has been measured to a certain extent by the oft-cited infant-mortality and longevity rates of the United States, which compare poorly to many other countries, despite the higher per capita income and investment in health in the USA. It seems clear that our health services industry produces its services inefficiently, at least when seen from the viewpoint of the whole society.

Three broad classifications of solutions are currently offered to these many problems: national health insurance (NHI), manpower programs, and reorganization of care. (A fourth classification, regional health planning, aims mainly at the cost factor, through macro rather than micro organizational changes.)

A. National Health Insurance (NHI)

NHI, which falls under the jurisdiction of the Senate Finance Committee and the House Ways and Means Committee, can be used to attack all three of the central issues in medical care—cost, equality, and appropriateness. Exactly how it is used for which of these issues will determine the relevance of NHI, as adopted, for the health problems of the migrants.

The issue of personal cost for health services will have to be addressed, since it is the most highly visible issue, and since NHI deals with finances intimately. The central idea of insurance, however, is not so much to control the social extent of cost as to control its personal predictability. That is, one buys insurance if he prefers a smaller certain loss to a larger uncertain one. Insurance is classically used to *spread* costs, *not decrease* them. In fact, if NHI includes poor groups—such as migrants—who currently do not receive much in the way of medical care, and who must receive transfer payments to participate in the program, costs will be *increased* to the middle and upper classes. Likewise, if NHI provides benefits without much control total costs will increase along with increased utilization. The temptation will therefore doubtless be present (1) to exclude poor groups from a significant amount of services, (2) to give NHI the *appearance* of saving money to the middle and upper classes, regardless of the real situation, as well as (3) to cut costs in a social sense by exercising certain controls.

Exclusion of poor groups from services can be effected in many ways. One way is to establish different programs for those with different income levels, and provide less coverage for the lower income groups. Another way is to establish a single program for all, but make mandatory coverage very slight and depend on voluntary coverage for the most part, so poor groups and those without sufficient leverage over their employers get poor coverage. A third way is to make enrollment cumbersome, with lots of red tape and discriminatory provisions (residency requirements, length of employment requirements, etc.), so that although on paper it appears almost all qualify, in fact many poor go uncovered. A fourth way is to include financial disincentives to use, such as high deductible and copayment features, that act preferentially against the poor, although some of these controls can sometimes have a positive control aspect. Clearly, each of these exclusionary tactics is a danger to the migrant. Most of these dangers would be shared by other poor groups. In reality, the complex issue of transfers–who pays how much for whom–is the central point of conflict in the NHI debate, even if it is often hidden.

NHI in various forms can rather easily be made to have the appearance of saving money. The benefits of medical care tend to be highly visible: medical care is a palpable service delivered on average five times annually to each American as an outpatient. As currently paid, health insurance and direct medical fees tend to be very visible as well. Simply decreasing the visibility of the latter–payments–should give the appearance of decreased personal cost for medical care. A major attraction of employer contribution-employee payroll deductions is the decreased visibility of payments, and the appearance to the worker of someone else's paying for him, although the worker often gives up possible wage increases to support that coverage. Financing from general revenues has the same, or even more pronounced effect. On the other hand, NHI could emphasize visible services at the expense of less visible but more important ones. The major danger here, to general public and migrant alike, is that apparent solutions to the real problem of cost control might replace substantial ones.

Real costs *can* be cut by an NHI program, and it is in fact the inability of the current system to control current cost trends that has made NHI an issue. That it is not clear that NHI will take significant steps to control real costs attests to the influence of the interests who benefit from the status quo in medical care. Reorganization of the current forms of medical practice, emphasis on preventive programs, control of hospital utilization, strong regional health facilities planning, and fee controls are only some of the mentioned controls that could be used. None of these would be counter-productive from the migrants point of view. Rather, it will be the efforts of "the interests" to divert efforts from real cost control to the two previously mentioned forms of spurious cost control (as well as to other issues), that will threaten the migrants.

NHI will also have to deal with the question of equality. The other side of the coin of equality is financial equity; the more migrants and other poor groups are included in richer benefit packages, the more other, wealthier Americans will have to pay for them, one way or another. Some amount of redistribution of cost is pretty much inevitable with NHI; any federal contributions must come from somewhere, and the choice of source will determine the type of cost redistribution. In addition, the choice of benefit packages and their distribution will affect the extent and the direction of the redistribution. The different possibilities of financing are complex and extensive in number and variation. Almost all things are possible, but the principles are clear. Reliance for financing on general revenues, derived mainly from progressive personal income tax and corporate taxes, or reliance on progressive or proportionate contributions specifically for NHI, would make for rich-to-poor transfers. Choices of large mandatory benefit packages would accentuate the transfer. Of course, regressive fund collections would decrease or possibly even reverse the transfer. Fragmentation of benefit packages would have the same effect, since those who could pay more would get more. As a have-not group, the migrants clearly have an interest in as great a transfer as possible—that is, financing by progressive means, and a high-level uniform benefit package.

NHI could also have an interesting secondary effort on equality. If NHI should be passed with sufficient strength to increase demand in undeserved areas, there would soon appear dissatisfaction among frustrated would-be patients and harried physicians alike. This pressure would then be a strong influence in producing stronger and more extensive programs for manpower production, redistribution, and medical care reorganization. Such possible consequences are well realized by government officials and legislators, and constitute a strong impediment to passage of NHI in any strong form.

The effects NHI would have on the appropriateness of care could vary greatly. There must be some effect, if only because the provisions of NHI will authorize only certain services, and will encourage some at the expense of others. For instance, the provisions of NHI will influence how much and what kind of preventive care, rehabilitative care, etc., are delivered; how many services will be performed outside and inside the hospital; and what the demand for different specialties and generalities will be. The provisions will also determine if prepayment alternatives are possible and attractive. These influences of NHI on appropriateness are mandatory. In addition, NHI legislation can go quite far into the field of organization with specific provisions for consciously thought out organizational objectives. For instance, many HMO objectives could be advanced in NHI legislation (see below), or quality review provision could be included. The migrants' interest would be served in this area pretty much as would the rest of the general public's, although more emphatically because of the usually more severe problems migrants have with appropriateness than the general public. That is, the financial barrier to health care having been cleared to a greater or lesser extent by inclusion of migrants in NHI coverage, the other barriers to care must be swept away as well. Care must be made purchasable, facilities and personnel must be present in the areas where the migrants are, the providers must be known to the migrants, and willing and able to accommodate them. Provisions in NHI that would promote establishment of group practices, increase the availability of primary practitioners in rural areas, etc., would make it very much easier for the migrants to be properly served. Since migrants need organized access to care in most instances, organized providers would be of special benefit to them. But, no matter how many "appropriateness" provisions were written into NHI, it is certain that all the special problems of the migrants—their isolation, language gaps, cultural gaps, etc.—would not be solved by them.

NHI could provide a great deal for the migrants, or on the other hand it could provide little of any real use. It depends primarily on how extensive the benefits are, and how many migrants are covered. Even if NHI were to solve none of the problems of appropriateness, and none of the cost problems, if the benefits were substantial and the migrants included in coverage, NHI would be of tremendous benefit to the migrants.

Financial barriers are extremely important in the migrants' exclusion from medical care. NHI could very significantly decrease these barriers, as no other realistically imaginable legislation would. Any program for migrant health must have a strong financial basis; NHI, with or without frills, is by far the best bet.

B. Manpower Programs

Like NHI, manpower programs can also be used to attack all three issues of cost, equality, and appropriateness. Unlike NHI, these programs are in most respects rather uncontroversial. And unlike NHI, manpower programs are currently operative in a form likely to be constant for some years. The forms are mainly the Comprehensive Health Manpower Training Act of 1971, the Nurse Training Act of 1971, and the Emergency Health Personnel Act, which established the National Health Service Corps (NHSC). Also included would be the Allied Health Professions Personnel Training Act, and the Health Improvement Act of 1970.

The effect of manpower programs on cost comes from two basic sources. First, as the supply of physicians and other personnel rises one would expect salaries to decrease and, correspondingly, unit costs. This effect is far from assured, however, since among other reasons, it seems unlikely from current projections that the physician supply increase would significantly increase competition. Also, many factors besides personnel charges affect the total price of medical care. In addition, the lag of effect should be at least eight to ten years.

More significant for cost reduction are efforts to train and employ intermediate level medical workers, and to use nurses for certain functions physicians usually perform. Both the CHMTA and NTA give substantial support for such efforts. The total effect should be enhanced productivity of the medical care system and lower cost for many services. Here, again, the impact of the programs should be a number of years in the future, particularly in light of restrictive state laws, insurance regulations, and entrenched custom.

Efforts to decrease personal costs by increasing medical manpower is basically not injurious to the interests of migrants and the rest of the poor. To some extent decreases in personal costs will be reflected in the national costs, especially with intermediate level personnel. Only if the latter were to be employed excessively, in a manner to decrease quality of care, would there be a deleterious effect, most likely on the migrant.

Manpower increase and voluntary redistribution is the least controversial means of promoting equality of medical care. Current programs hope that by increasing personnel supply by health school financing and intermediate level personnel training, the increased medical care capacity will have a chance to spill over to currently undercovered regions. Thus will equality increase while no one's care will be impaired. Such an effect, if it comes, is bound to be long range.

The Comprehensive Health Manpower Training Act of 1971 also has provisions for loan forgiveness in return for work in primary care in needy areas (the Nurse Training Act also forgives loans for nurses who work in areas with a shortage of and need for nurses), and there is even a provision, (Sec. 784) inserted by the Senate, for scholarships to medical students who promise to work for a number of years in a physician shortage area, or an area where they will care for a substantial number of migrant workers. These voluntary redistribution programs have been tried before in many states, and unfortunately generally do not work. Most loan or scholarship recipients choose to buy their way out of their obligations after their training has been completed. The scholarship grant program might have better luck than usual, since it specifies preference for individuals of low income coming from needy areas themselves. But, in any event, the time lag is likely to be at least eight to ten years. One further provision of the Comprehensive Health Manpower Training Act of 1971 designed to help equalize medical care might prove of some help in the near future. The Act calls for establishment in HEW of a National Health Manpower Shortage Clearinghouse, charged with the function of "provid(ing) information to, and maintain(ing) listings of, (1) communities and areas with health professional needs, and (2) prospective health workers interested in such opportunities." This effort could well be of great help to the MHP in recruiting.

Finally, another provision of the same act calls for the Secretary of HEW to "use his best efforts to provide, to each county certified by him to be without the services of a physician physically residing within such county, at least one physician in the Public Health Service, except for counties so sparsely populated as not to require such a physician." This provision will be of little or no help to migrants, since such areas are few, and not migrant areas, anyway.

More direct and more immediate than the Comprehensive Health Manpower Training Act of 1971 is the Emergency Health Personnel Act, fathered mainly by Senator Warren Magnuson, chairman of the HEW Appropriations Subcommittee. This Act established a National Health Service Corps, which can employ physicians and others as PHS officers, give them credit for military service to count against the draft, and assign them to areas of medical need in the country. For the near future, the lawmakers are relying on the NHSC to fill some of the gaps of care in poor areas.

Although it is clear many of the personnel could be used in migrant areas, there are obvious shortcomings in the law. The persons to be employed are in a sense to do missionary work, denying themselves the rewards they could find in the marketplace. Missionary medicine is not compatible with a sense of dignity of the receivers. Secondly, the duration of time spent by the physician would be rather short, a handicap in administering continuous care. Thirdly, since the attractiveness of the NHSC is at present predicated on the existence of the doctor draft, and since the doctor draft is ending, the attractiveness of the program will be in doubt. Fourthly, since the law necessitates endorsement by the local medical society of an area where personnel will be provided, it is likely that many areas with need and a regressive and competitive medical society will be denied that endorsement. Fifthly, because of that endorsement requirement, it is unlikely that progressive methods of organization or competitive amenities would be associated with the services provided. Sixthly, it is unlikely that physicians on the federal payroll would be well accepted by the surrounding medical community, especially since the tenor of the NHSC encourages "idealists" to apply, and those "idealists" would be just the ones most likely to antagonize the local medical community. The viability of the local programs would often be in doubt, therefore. Seventhly, anyone familiar with the past actions of organized medicine has difficulty visualizing its allowing for long a substantial federal effort to supply quality medicine to undersupplied areas in anything like the necessary amount. Finally, the federal administrators, at least under the present administration, are unlikely to emphasize the program much. They opposed its passage and significantly delayed its implementation after passage, placing it in an inconspicuous part of the Community Health Service. Realizing the inherent conflict with local, private medicine, they are unlikely to risk much on this, to their eyes, low priority program.

On the other hand, it is possible that many of these problems will be avoided or minimized. Along with the end of the draft is scheduled to come a substantial increase of salaries for medical officers that will presumably apply to the PHS. The missionary aspect will thereby be ameliorated and recruiting aided. The increasingly patient-centered orientation of some young health workers and their rising idealism might also serve to fill the NHSC ranks. Transience need not be a major hazard if proper organizational arrangements can be made. It is also possible for the role of the local medical societies to be curtailed.

Although all these variables make the general future and significance of the NHSC problematic, its significance for the MHP should not be underestimated. Attracting physicians, and in some cases other personnel, to MHP projects seemed to be a problem before the NHSC; the national recruiting apparatus and publicity attendant to the NHSC should increase the pool of physicians available greatly. Not only that, but if NHSC personnel staff MHP projects, extra money will in effect be transferred to the MHP. NHSC personnel working under non-MHP auspices might also be in a position to help many migrants. In the future, if substantial organized migrant health medical care facilities are established in many areas, it might be possible to rotate these personnel through the various centers as patient loads change throughout the seasons. Particularly if centers develop that treat resident populations extensively as well as migrants, NHSC personnel could prove a key ingredient to the "accordion" model of care (one that expands and contracts services according to demand in a regular fashion). In the near future, however, given the recent controversiality of the MHP, only very few personnel can be expected to be assigned to MHP projects from the NHSC.

The manpower programs also attempt to affect the appropriateness of care. Through grants, contracts, loans, scholarships, and such, the recent Acts seek to support training in family medicine and the team approach to the provision of health services, adoption of the computer in routine medical care, training of intermediate level personnel, etc. The ultimate effect of these provisions is not readily predictable, but the lag time before they are felt will surely be appreciable. Moreover, even with the multiple provisions seeking to redistribute care, it is most likely that effects will first take place around the academic institutions where the programs will be housed, and only later will the innovations diffuse out to the provinces, and the migrants. When and if they do reach the migrants, however, the innovations will be helpful.

The manpower programs, then, will affect migrant health, but not profoundly. The manpower legislation approaches cost benignly, seeking to increase manpower, especially in primary care, and to promote use of intermediate level personnel, hoping prices will be stabilized by a larger input and increased productivity on the supply side. This approach to cost stabilization is not threatening to the migrants; it is an approach that attempts to get at the root of part of the cost problem, rather than deliver less care to the poor. The manpower bills likewise attempt to equalize care in a benign if not immediately effective way. It is hoped that increased productivity and input on the supply side will spill over to the needy areas, encouraged by voluntary measures such as some limited financial incentives, educational approaches, coordination approaches, and voluntary service with the best hope for the migrants to get service delivered in the near future, although there are doubts as to whether they will get them or not. The other measures are likely to be of some value, but not until the next decade. This very soft approach might be considered threatening to the migrants in that some might think that a great deal is being done herewith to help them, when in fact it amounts to doing just that which will be offensive to no one. The manpower approaches have some effects on appropriateness also, but the lag time will be very long.

In sum, the long-range manpower approaches will benefit the migrants eventually by increasing the rural medical capacity factor, but by how much is problematic. The more immediately applicable program, NHSC, will possibly serve to make medical care available soon for some more migrants, but there are some strong questions about its political strength.

C. Reorganization of Medical Care—Health Maintenance Organizations

The third major medical care issue now being considered is that of medical care reorganization.[c] NHI could well be used for impetus in medical care reorganization, and provisions in NHI will affect the extent and type of reorganization. Likewise, the health manpower programs will have a bearing on what kind of reorganization is possible, since organization must be adapted to the numbers and types of personnel available, and to their training. But whereas the issue of organization lies rather latent in each of those programs, in governmental encouragement of so-called Health Maintenance Organizations, the issue of reorganization is considered in its manifest form.

The idea of prepaid group practice has been advocated by medical care liberals for many years; during the Kennedy-Johnson years the efforts in this direction took second place to equality as the fight for Medicare was underway. Later, the issue of organization came more clearly into focus, in combination with the issue of equality, as money was allocated for health programs for the poor cast in new organizational forms—chiefly in neighborhood health centers. Reorganization at a higher level was also stimulated by regional planning programs. With the Nixon Administration, the trend to emphasize reorganization and de-emphasize equality has found expression in the HMO legislative and administrative initiatives.

An HMO is explained as having four parts to it. The first is the health delivery system of personnel and facilities, the second is an enrolled population,

[c]The Health Maintenance Organization Act of 1973 was signed into law on December 29, 1973. The conference report stated that, "the purpose of this legislation is to stimulate greater provider and consumer interest in and awareness of the HMO concept of health care delivery. This is to be achieved through a combination of financial assistance and improved access to potential markets." Setting a priority for underserved areas and a 20% set-aside of funds for rural areas, the Act authorizes $25 million for fiscal year 1974, $55 million for 1975, and $85 for 1976 and 1977. The Act's general approach is to authorize grants and contracts for feasibility surveys; grants, contracts, and loan guarantees for planning and for initial developments costs; and loans and loan guarantees for initial operation costs. The original Senate version of the legislation specifically authorized the support of HMO's for migrants under the MHP, but the final version (taking note of the House MHP legislation then under development) authorizes support if funds other than MHP funds are utilized. The results of this entitlement are not yet clear.

the third is a financial plan whereby the enrolled population prepays a set amount of money and is accordingly entitled to certain services from the personnel and facilities, and the fourth is management of this system. Different degrees of "tightness" of organization are envisioned, from the relatively tight Kaiser model to the relatively loose San Joaquin Medical Care Foundation model. HMOs incorporate the basic ideas of traditional prepaid-group practice.

The legislation envisioned, much like the manpower legislation, is incentive, voluntary legislation, rather than mandatory legislation. Different proposals call for grants and contracts for planning and development, insurance options, educational initiatives, legal enabling legislation, grants to cover initial costs, grants and loans for construction, and grants and contracts for methodological development.

The objectives of HMOs can be described in terms of the three basic rubrics we have been using, cost, equality, and appropriateness. Cost control is a prime objective. At the micro level, the cost impact of HMOs might well be significant, because of altered incentives and improved productivity. Each HMO enrollee should feel this effect. The problem of transfers to poor patients must be faced, however; as with NHI, if poor patients are to be provided with services they were previously denied, even if cost per patient is to drop, cost per *paying* patient may rise. This contingency can be avoided by excluding the poor from benefits (unlikely) or minimized by limiting their benefits (likely). Individual costs to the paying patient can also be concealed by drawing the poor patients' enrollment fees from general revenues or perhaps the central Social Security fund. Exactly how this is managed will be important.

Societal costs are also contained by HMOs. Since the financial connection between the government and the medical care providers is so simple, HMOs can "improv(e) (the) ability of Federal and State programs to control their health care expenditures with predictable prepaid contracts for beneficiaries."[5] The key role of government in controlling societal cost and expenditure levels through HMOs thus becomes apparent—some assert cogently that it is precisely this possibility which attracts the current administration so strongly to HMOs. Another social cost benefit of HMOs is that by increasing the centralization of medical care, possibilities for central planning are improved.

HMOs can affect equality only passively. Since HMOs are not a source of financing in themselves, the most an HMO bill could do would be to include provisions to ensure an HMO would not discriminate, except on a financial basis. The flexibility of an HMO would be able to accommodate whatever financing scheme is arrived at nationally (or otherwise), since different benefit packages could apply to different groups. In the specific amenities offered to different types of enrollees, such as the respect accorded to each, the HMOs could vary, depending on the organization, personnel, and other factors.

HMOs stand to be very effective in appropriateness of care delivered. Much of the argument favoring group practice has concerned just this subject.

Theoretically, accessibility, availability, acceptability, continuity, and comprehensiveness of care can be greatly enhanced, although much depends on the specific administrative set-up employed. Quality and quality control can be enhanced, and full utilization of paramedical personnel is encouraged. Delivery of preventive care is encouraged as well.

Migrants can benefit from these elements of appropriateness as well as anyone, of course, as long as they have access to them. Of particular benefit is the element of easy accessibility, which makes it much easier for the transient migrant to find care. The HMO falls into the same pattern of organization as the health center idea put forward in Chapter 3.

Technically, then, HMOs seem well suited to deal with cost and appropriateness of medical care, standing neutral on the issue of equality. The migrants stand to benefit from HMOs, but only if they are dealt in financially. It would be a good way of avoiding the possibility of second-rate care, in fact, if the migrants could be enrolled by special contract into various HMOs along their route, and have these HMOs equipped with special outreach capabilities, plus other capabilities of relevance to the migrants, if possible.

While HMOs harbor technical promise for migrants, the political outlook is more foreboding. As pointed out above, the big administration push for HMOs, as opposed to its cautious approach toward NHI and manpower programs, betokens an outlook that objects to further financial encumbrances. In other words, the trend away from supporting equalizing programs to supporting programs of cost control and increased appropriateness eliminates precisely that element the migrants need most. Such a move can be made to sound good: ". . . the poor should not bear the brunt of supporting innovation in health care delivery."[6] But in fact, in 1971 HSMHA took money formerly devoted to medical care for the poor in the Partnership for Health program, and reallocated it to large companies for HMO planning and development. So, while HMOs might be technically neutral on the question of equality, politically they can be anti-equalitarian.

Unlike the situation with NHI, where the Senate Finance Committee and House Ways and Means Committee hold jurisdiction, HMOs fall under the Labor and Public Welfare Committee and Interstate and Foreign Commerce Committee. As noted, these latter committees are likely to be more receptive to migrant and equalizing entreaties than the former. The leverage obtained by refusing HMO legislation, or including equalizing provisions (as far as these are possible without financing), however, is not likely to be decisive.

D. Summary and Implications

Medical care policy developments center around three basic non-unanimous societal demands: cost control, equality of services to all, and increased appropriateness of medical care arrangements. Three different governmental efforts are being currently proposed to deal with these questions: national health insurance (NHI), manpower development, and reorganization through health maintenance organizations (HMO). The effects of the programs on the societal demands would be as follows: *NHI* will probably control costs by some combination of not including the poor fully, hiding payments and displaying benefits, and decreasing unit costs. It must certainly increase the equality of medical services delivered, but to an adjustable extent. Effects on the appropriateness of care could vary widely.

The *manpower* programs passed will probably eventually aid in decreasing unit costs by increasing the supply of all personnel, and particularly intermediate level personnel. They will contribute to equality of care by increasing the supply of personnel to the point where a spillover to underserved populations occurs, by directly influencing personnel to serve in poorly served areas, by directly assigning personnel to poorly served areas through the National Health Service Corps, and by coordinating needy areas and willing personnel through a clearinghouse. Appropriateness of services will also probably be eventually improved by training in areas such as family and team medicine.

HMOs will probably be able to decrease unit service costs and costs per person by utilizing group practice and prepayment; exclusion of the poor from coverage could decrease total societal costs. Control of societal and governmental expenditures would be much facilitated by HMOs. The question of equality is hit only obliquely by HMOs. The big question would be who would be included in the HMOs, a financing question; after inclusion, equal or unequal treatment for different groups would depend on the HMO administration. HMOs would hit quite directly on appropriateness, contributing to accessibility, availability, continuity, quality, etc.

The central issue in NHI is equality—who is going to get financed for what. The central thrust in HMOs is cost control and appropriateness of services. The manpower programs are in a sense a prerequisite for the other two—neither will be successful without the proper manpower input. If NHI were to be passed, it would need many of the elements of HMOs—to control costs, and to organize care so that it would be purchasable. That is why some of the most thoughtful NHI proposals contain HMO elements. On the other hand, HMOs do not need NHI—they could do well working on the same financial base that is found at present, and avoid the issue of equality.

The degree of political controversy of these programs follows from the above assertions. The manpower legislation has been relatively uncontroversial except in its financial aspects, the administration delaying implementation significantly. Basically, increasing manpower seems to take nothing away from anyone. HMOs have been moderately controversial, the main implications of the proposals being unclear. Most opposition has come from the private physician sector and from those who fear that focusing on HMOs obscures the issue of equality. NHI is highly controversial and highlights a basic internal conflict in the American value system, pitting as it does the value of equality against that of financial equity.

IV CONSEQUENCES OF HEALTH CARE POLICY FOR MIGRANTS AND THE MIGRANT HEALTH PROGRAM

This section will examine to what extent NHI, manpower, and HMO legislation would solve the health problems of the migrants, consider what needs would be missed, and suggest what supplemental actions could be taken specifically on the migrants' behalf.

A. Contributions of New Health Policy to Migrant Health

To find out how NHI, manpower programs, and HMOs would affect the migrants, let us assume that all are passed in a form that includes the migrants in coverage, and are fairly strong measures. Then, just as in Chapter 3, let us review the causality chart of migrant poor health with reference to the effects that would be found. As before, the rankings of effects must be estimates, and even more unsatisfactory than before, since we are dealing with an unknown configuration of programs. Still, the general profile will be of interest.

1. Poverty (0). The impoverished state of migrants would be ameliorated only to the extent that money for the purchase of medical care would be available. Although this in itself is to some extent an antipoverty effect, by convention we give this effect a rating of zero. The non-medical care precursors to poor health would not be much ameliorated by personal funds now freed up by not having to pay for medical care.

2. Mobility (++). NHI by its national character (probably) would make medical care purchasable anywhere a provider could be found, and would therefore be helpful in countering the effects of mobility. HMOs could make a contribution also, by providing an organizational focus of comprehensive services that would improve accessibility. The National Health Service Corps, especially if members were to be rotated to different centers according to the season, would also be helpful. Still needed, however, would be special outreach efforts to make medical care truly accessible to the migrants, as well as stream coordination of records and services. The effect of mobility on environmental variables—housing, sanitation—would not be improved. Also unaffected would be the psychological effects that migrancy itself has on children and families.

3. Discrimination (++). Several effects to counter discrimination could be expected. If NHSC personnel should be used, their motivation in dealing with migrants might often be quite positive. Likewise with the personnel recruited from poor, rural areas and given loans to attend health professional school, when

they serve in poor areas to gain loan forgiveness. HMOs might be useful to integrate the migrant means of care and the general means of care. NHI might have a similar effect, and might give the migrants a minor voice in the private marketplace, despite the many barriers. The fact that NHI and HMO programs would be widely based, with migrants participating on an equal basis with all, would also accrue to the migrants' benefit.

On the other side of the question, however, there would be little possibility or incentive to employ migrants or similar socioeconomic groups as workers in the systems. Nor would there be much possibility of including migrants in informational feedback systems, and certainly not direct participation in design and control of the systems. Finally, much of the profound prejudice found in society that affects not only medical care provision, but other health affecting categories such as housing, environment, and occupational conditions would be left unaffected.

4. Rural Medical Capacity (++). NHI could provide for redistribution of resources, and for reorganization and increased productivity of those resources. Such provisions are quite unlikely to materialize, however, and the major effect NHI will have on rural medical care capacity would be the small one of more evenly dividing the financial incentives for medical services among different areas of the country. As pointed out before, however, money does not seem to be the answer to redistribution. The manpower programs will have positive, if mostly long-range and rather weak, effects. The programs count on a spillover to needy areas as a result of a general increase in the supply of manpower, redistribution as a specific effect of financial incentives, increased productivity to all areas from increased use of new types of personnel in teams, and finally an immediate effect on poor areas through direct assignment of teams of personnel assigned to the National Health Service Corps. HMOs should have a positive effect by increasing productivity.

The limitation of these attacks is that they are permissive, voluntary measures, rather than strong, mandatory ones. None of the proposed measures likely to pass will take anything away from "them what's got." A definitive measure would be an "underserved area bill" to produce manpower for underserved areas in a short period of time, of necessity decreasing the supply in currently well served areas, and to organize care in those underserved areas. Such a bill would be an important development.

5. Environment (0). No effect.

6. Occupation (0). No effect.

7. Nutrition (0). No effect.

8. Medical Care (+++). All the current health efforts aim at the delivery of health care, and to the extent that migrants are included in the benefits proposed, to the extent those benefits are comprehensive, and to the extent availability and accessibility problems are solved, medical care will be delivered. There are many unknowns here; unlike the programs mentioned in

Chapter 3, the migrants are not the major target of legislation in these general health measures, and it is quite possible for the migrants to receive but little. Furthermore, the need for outreach to overcome many barriers to care for the migrants and the need for coordination of care along the stream are not met by these programs. Nonetheless, especially in the case of NHI and the NHSC, immediate provision of medical care is the air, and NHI provides the most crucial impediment of all, money.

8a. Type of Care (+++). The quality and extensiveness of care offered will be, once again, greatly dependent on the terms of NHI. The manpower programs aim at producing more care without a drop in quality, and the NHSC should employ young but qualified practitioners in primary care, probably in less than adequate organizational settings. HMOs would promote appropriateness of care, and would decrease the possibility of two-class medicine. Especially in the short run, the lack of adequate manpower (quality and quantity) in rural areas will make the quality of care delivered low. Furthermore, the permissiveness of the HMO legislation allows loose configurations that would not necessarily be conducive to high quality care and qualitative review. But assuming the widespread application of HMOs, the type of care offered migrants should be pretty good.

9. Efficiency (+++). NHI would probably avoid many of the usual insurance inefficiencies, and HMOs would lead to improved productivity. Moreover, manpower programs that emphasize intermediate level professional development would also make an efficiency contribution. A point of inefficiency would be undue concentration on medical care provision without balancing efforts on other precursors of poor health.

10. Spillover (0). No extra jobs would be offered migrants, no political uplift, etc.

The assessment results can be summarized as follows:

poverty	*mobility*	*discrimination*	*rural med. capacity*	*environment*
0	++	++	++	0

occupation	*nutrition*	*medical care*	*type of care*	*efficiency*	*spillover*
0	0	+++	+++	+++	0

This is not so bad a record, especially considering the profiles of the alternative programs listed in Chapter 3. This good record demonstrates, in fact, how much the health problems of migrants resemble those of other Americans, for these programs that turn out to help the migrants significantly are aimed at the general population. We have assumed ideal programs, however, in the assessment. Mere passage of NHI faces formidable hurdles, and promoting HMOs on more than an experimental basis is problematic as well.

Our approach here, however, should point out two things: one, if NHI and HMOs were put into effect, along with the already approved manpower programs, their contributions to the health of migrants could be substantial; and two, even if all were to be passed in fairly idealized form, there would still be many uncovered facets to the migrant ill health causality scheme.

It is profitable to look at what still would be needed for the health of migrants if NHI, manpower programs, and HMOs all were put into effect at generous levels. (If those programs were not passed, or were passed with less than ideal provisions, to the following list could simply be added those elements missing from the legislation.)

First and foremost, the overall problem of poverty would have to be attacked. This problem lies beyond the range of this report.

Second, accessibility to medical care would have to be assured by outreach programs designed to reach migrants both upstream and downstream. Registration for insurance would have to be accomplished through impetus by others than the individual, isolated migrant–excessive red tape and other barriers to registration are often relied on to keep utilization down.

Third, something would have to be done to prevent the migrancy itself from causing ill effects. Most likely many of these effects are unavoidable as long as the migrant way of life persists. Still, efforts to minimize the extent of migrancy required, by a humanistic ordering of the labor cycle, for instance, instead of the chaotic competition, uncertainty, and frenetic movement found, would contribute to improvement of psycho-social conditions and consequently mental health.

Fourth, the problem of discrimination would have to be handled in such a way that migrants were not only guaranteed full access to acceptable medical care, which could be handled through outreach programs connected to HMOs and the NHSC, but also so that discrimination did not express itself in poor housing conditions, substandard working conditions, etc.

Fifth, the current approaches to manpower redistribution are too weak to work. Capacity to produce medical care in rural areas will therefore remain insufficient. Specific recruitment for migrant care would be indicated.

Sixth, the environmental problems would still have to be attacked. These can be attacked both at the local level, through enforcement of regulations, self-help, and pressure and persuasion, and at state and federal levels, with passage of protective laws and programs for environmental improvement.

Seventh, the problem of occupation would still have to be attacked. Since field work in itself is probably enough to be unduly hard on a person's health, opportunities for leaving the line of work should be supplied. Efforts to reduce occupational hazards and improve working conditions should also be made.

Eighth, specific efforts to improve nutrition must be made, by providing money, food stamps, or commodities.

Ninth, surveillance to monitor the health of migrants would be necessary, for it would be a clear tendency in general programs such as those under consideration to forget the powerless migrants.

From those nine points it seems clear that, despite passage of these three medical care programs, the need for additional aid would still exist. Concentrating on medical care, the programs miss all the elements of poor health causation that do not have to do with medical care—environment, occupation, etc. In addition, the medical care measures do not even cover all the elements necessary for medical care delivery—outreach and personnel redistribution, for example. Clearly, if the MHP was to sponsor regional health centers, many of the neglected functions would be served. Further, the idealized provisions envisioned here are unlikely to come to reality, and functions postulated as being fulfilled by NHI or HMOs would have to be taken over by a special program for migrants.

B. How the MHP Could Anticipate Health Policy Developments

Chapter 3 found the regional health center approach in many ways the most appropriate. Not considered were problems such as start-up costs, lag time until fruition, and the relative merits of different phase-in methods; only end-points were judged. The basic principle for introducing regional health centers to the MHP, so as to best adjust to NHI and HMOs, should now be derived.

It does seem fairly clear what the end-point should look like. There should be, according to Chapter 3, a system of regional health centers, concentrating first on high-impact migrant areas, organized for the community at large as well as the migrants with such funds and other aid as might be available from HMO-promoting agencies, supported through patient payments with NHI, using personnel made available directly and indirectly through the manpower legislation, and equipped with special necessary migrant provisions, such as outreach, environmental and occupational improvement capabilities, etc.

In deciding how to get to this end-point, the following conditions should be observed:

1. A proper balance should be found between providing services in the present and preparing for the future, so that the value of the time-stream of services provided is maximized. In other words, the MHP should expedite proper use of NHI and HMO funds for migrants when they become available, but not sacrifice an excessive amount of present services to do it. No exact solution to this problem will or can be found, but approximations should be possible as choices present themselves.
2. A proper balance should be found between the risk one takes by having MHP strategy deviate from its optimum if there were to be no interaction with any other program, and the probabilities of passage and provisions of NHI and HMOs. In other words, if we knew for sure when NHI and HMOs would come and what they would entail, we could plan accordingly without risk. If we knew they were not coming at all, we could do likewise. Given, however, only vague probabilities of both time and contents, one must pay close attention

to the risks involved and weigh them against probable payoffs. As always, payoffs should be counted strictly for the migrant and agricultural workers, not others, such as all rural residents, or health professionals.

3. The chance to integrate health services for migrants and the general populace should be maximized, although necessary ancillary services for migrants should not be lost.
4. The continuing development of solutions for particular problems—ways of attacking the non-medical care problems especially—should be maximized.
5. The need for special migrant provisions in addition to general medical care programs should be well illustrated.
6. The strategy adopted should be compatible with the staff capabilities of the MHP, whether changed or static.

Theoretically, it is extremely difficult to deal with so many interacting requirements, even disregarding the fact that other requirements at different levels and of different significance could also be added. Practically speaking, perhaps because he believes that it is extremely important to be concrete in detailing any plans and because he is very suspicious that lack of clarity will redound to the disadvantage of the migrant, the author can assert only two reasonable basic strategies that the MHP could wisely follow in the near future. These two strategies can be rated against the above requirements and then compared. Other strategies can be imagined—one would be concentration on just those elements that would not be covered by NHI and HMOs—outreach, coordination along the stream, etc. All those strategies that the author can think of, however, are so quickly disposed of by rating against the requirements that it does not seem worthwhile to go through the mechanics here.

The two strategies can be called the "core" strategy and the "full scale" strategy. The "core" strategy would entail the MHP's setting up "core" services—a minimum possible "critical mass" of the regional health center model—in as many areas as possible, so that when NHI money became available, those "cores" could act as organizing principals that would grow to provide all necessary services. The "full scale" strategy would entail establishment of regional health centers in various areas and full development of their potential until they covered all the migrants (and agricultural workers) in the area for all their health needs.

The *first criterion* to judge on is service-now versus service-in-the-future. The "core" strategy is specifically tailored to emphasize the latter, the "full scale" strategy the former. Not only would the "core" strategy provide many niduses for immediate application of NHI funds, but the practice obtained by the MHP staff in setting up such projects would enable them to do all the better when NHI came to be enacted. Furthermore, use could be made of the limited funds presently available for HMO development. Clearly, however, these advantages would be obtained with a cost to present care. Start-up costs would be incurred repeatedly, and possible economies of scale would not be reached. Also, the possibility for individual continued dynamism in projects (most often dependent on growth) would be denied, and might compromise the viability of many projects.

The "full scale" strategy would maximize the current service payoff, as determined previously, with full access to exploiting growth potential. There might be points reached at which diseconomies of scale set in, as with trying to reach very difficult patients, which would tend to negate the size advantage, but it would be possible to limit growth to lesser amounts in those cases. Likewise, start-up costs would be incurred to a minimal extent, also contributing to maximizing current payoff. Currently available HMO money might be used for development of these systems, perhaps even to the same extent as in the "core" strategy, since advanced system development could be covered. With the advent of NHI the "full scale" approach would not be providing immediate help to migrants in spending that money properly and usefully. The process of starting up new projects would have to begin from scratch in many areas, and the rate of development would necessarily have to be very speedy. Furthermore, because of this delay, patterns for spending this new money might develop in the meantime that would be hard to erase once the organized center were in working condition. However, an advantage of the "full scale" approach relative to the response to NHI could be development of experienced personnel in the relatively mature centers that could move to new projects and contribute mightily to their development.

The *second criterion* on which to evaluate the services is risk and the uncertainty of the national programs. The "core" strategy clearly deviates from current optimum strategy without reference to NHI in hopes of a windfall in the near future. The risk is reduced by the fact that, even were NHI not to pass, more money allocated directly to the MHP could be expected to fill the gaps. Essentially, this approach would constitute a hedge, since if NHI money were still expected imminently, the additional MHP money would be spent for more new starts. The extent of the risk is also dependent on the definition of "core" accepted, since the more it deviated from "full scale," which would presumably be optimal, the more present services would be sacrificed.

The "full scale" strategy, on the other hand, is in essence the optimum strategy to be followed if only a slow and rather steady growth of resources for migrant health would be expected. The risk involved here would be that of lost opportunity were NHI to be passed and arrangements for migrant use of that money to be incomplete. One cannot call "core" or "full scale" more "risky" than the other without knowing the probabilities of NHI passage.

The *third criterion* calls for maximizing the possibility of achieving an integrated medical care delivery system in an area. This is a complicated question. It would seem most likely that if a system were set up initially to serve migrants, there would be a great deal of trouble converting that to an integrated system, because the stigma of the migrants would prevent others from wanting to be included. Even if the services for migrants were clearly superior to those the rest of the community could expect, chances are others would be quite hesitant to join, and chances are that migrant services would not long remain superior to the rest, given the basic discrepancy in power. On the other hand, given services that were developed with the intention of being integrated, the chances for migrants receiving services equal to those given others, especially with the need for special migrant services such as outreach, would also be less than 100 percent. Conflicts of interest between permanent population and migrants would tend to be decided in favor of the former; it would be difficult to build in an appropriate migrant voice. Given this dilemma, however, it would seem that integration from the beginning with due attention to migrant representation at decision-making levels would be the best bet.

The "core" strategy in this respect has the obvious disadvantage of starting many projects with only the migrants in mind. Developing an integrated system later on would be most likely accomplished by amalgamation of the "migrant core" into a more comprehensive system serving others as well. The only advantage of having started with the "core," then, would have been to start the organizing process of migrants around the issue of health. That is, migrants might be better able to represent themselves in the new integrated system than they would have before. It would also be possible, of course, for a "core" service to be started not just for migrants but for all in the community, by joint funding the initial effort with HMO or other money. In that case, the "core" strategy would not deter integrated systems, but rather encourage them.

The "full scale" strategy would in most instances not be able to promote integrated systems, since joint funding would be hard to come by. On the other hand, since the "full scale" projects would of necessity be located in fewer areas than the "core" projects, more areas would be free to start an integrated system from scratch at the introduction of NHI. Furthermore, the obvious high quality of the systems established would supply a better chance for integration of others while retaining the essentials of the established system, than would a "core" set up, which would be much more likely to lose its identity by being absorbed into another set up. Thus, where a "full scale" system were integrated, the migrants would be much more likely to remain top priority than where a "core" system were integrated.

The *fourth criterion* deals with continually developing solutions for problems. The "full scale" strategy would be an excellent avenue to pursue such efforts, but the "core" strategy would not be able to give sufficient resources to projects to let such attempts be made, nor would "core" projects have the institutional bulk to make such efforts fit into the projects properly. In this respect, then, the "full scale" strategy provides an option for being more future-productive than the "core" strategy.

The *fifth criterion* states that vivid illustration should be given of the special problems of the migrants and solutions to them. The intent here is to ensure that continued attention and support be directed the migrants even after passage of NHI. Since most of the investment in the "core" approach would be in start up efforts, the results of which would not be readily visible, and the more visible developments would be postponed, and the unique approaches to particularly migrant problems also postponed, the "core" approach would fare less well than "full scale" approach by this criterion.

Finally, the *sixth criterion* states that the efforts called for in the strategy adopted be consonant with the governmental personnel called upon to do the job. The "core" approach would call for a great deal of rather sophisticated governmental efforts—project initiation on a broad scale with sensitivity to local situations, exercise of flexibility and discretion, etc. Although such activities would be beyond the capabilities of the present staff, it might be possible to recruit an appropriate staff with this exciting mission in mind. As stated before, however, the difficulties of doing so would be substantial.

The "full scale" strategy also calls for a federal staff more skilled and creative than that found at present, but smaller than and with some skills different from the staff needed for the "core" strategy. The "full scale" strategy implies fewer centers, with not necessarily more work per center for federal staff, hence a lower federal manpower requirement. Some new starts would be made, so abilities to initiate local action would be needed. Since development of centers to the apex of their capabilities would be the largest charge, however, medical care administration ability and other abilities to help develop the necessary new approaches would be needed. Perhaps the requirements for the "full scale" approach would be somewhat less, because more might be left to local efforts. Still, it would seem to be just as hard to recruit able people for the "full scale" approach as for the "core" approach.

With the advent of NHI, both kinds of expertise—local project initiation and project systems development—would be needed, so it would be difficult to say which strategy would be more helpful in personnel development.

In summing up the distinctions between the two proposed strategies, it must first be stressed that they are really different points on a spectrum. The "core" approach looks at all locals in parallel, calling for initial development of as many areas as possible right away, and looks forward to a steady wave of advancement fueled by a timely infusion of NHI money. The "full scale" strategy adopts a series rather than parallel approach, calling for continually increasing support of projects until they reach their full potential in an area, starting other projects afterwards. This strategy would adapt to NHI when and if it comes by using NHI money to support a large part of its already established projects, and using its own resources to start new projects that would then continue to develop in the ways pioneered by the program before, with due allowance for individual variations. A mixed "core" and "full scale" strategy is possible and probable. Both strategies agree with the basic precept that when NHI money becomes available, it should be used to form the organizational basis.

How one defines the "core" of services also determines how far apart the two strategies lie. It would seem reasonable that the quality of care rendered must not be compromised, for once a facility is in the habit of dispensing a certain quality of care, and people are used to receiving it, it is difficult to change that habit. Furthermore, if adequate quality is not delivered, the value of the product becomes low very quickly. Since "quality" involves not only accuracy but extent as well, comprehensiveness of services is a must. Following this line of argument, the "core" of services runs up to beyond the $400,000-$500,000 per year projects funded in 1970. And that figure did not support any significant environmental efforts!

A major alternative to the "full scale" approach that avoided the possibility of excessive compromise on quality would be "cores" that consisted only of planning and organization, with no service. This extreme approach was one of those deemed not worthy of referring to the rating process, since a moment's thought quickly rules out this approach on almost all points (although one or two such grants with a view to immediate development might be worthwhile as part of the series approach). As soon as one breaks into services, however, system balance and minimum components as listed elsewhere (e.g., need for at least several physicians, which implies a need for many nurses, etc.) run the "core" up to a good deal of money.

The "full scale" projects would vary in total cost according to services offered and population covered, but one should be able to figure that a full project's population will have as much spent on it per person as the average person in the USA spends for health care each year—plus amounts for environmental services. A rough estimate of comparable sizes of "full scale" and "core" projects would then be about two or three to one in major migrant concentration areas.

Even if the two strategies are in many ways rather alike, what would their relative values be, if we were forced to choose? Listed by criteria, on #1 there was a standoff; #2 depended on NHI's chances at any given moment, and tilted toward "full scale"; #3 favored "full scale" generally, as did #4 and #5; and #6 was a standoff. "Full scale" is then a winner, but with the clear indication that a combination with the "core" strategy to salvage the latter's advantages (e.g., using HMO money to start new centers for integrated populations) should be established.

Determining how to combine the two strategies in practice is a fine opportunity for creative administration. As NHI looks more imminent and its details clearer, more new starts should be made. Opportunism with regard to local areas should be exercised: appearance of a strong consumer group, or expression of enlightened provider interest, or a favorable congressional situation should be exploited. Availability of HMO money most be weighed in. The personnel that can be recruited for the programs would have individual characteristics that would also effect formulation of proper program strategy. Some of these unpredictable events might even indicate the desirability on occasion of deviating from the regional health center approach, for instance, in some very important but refractory counties.

Manpower programs have not been mentioned so far in this section as a factor to be considered in formulating strategy, but the implications are fairly clear. Personnel are even now potentially available for migrant health activities from the National Health Service Corps, and will later be available from the loan forgiveness program. Places for employment of such persons should be identified, and the personnel claimed in behalf of the migrants.

Finally, just as it was clear in the chapter on administration, so it now should be clear that the MHP personnel and organization as presently constituted is for the most part unable to meet the creativity-demanding tasks set forth. Health policy developments and their implications for migrant health policy support the recommendation for MHP reorganization or special conditions within the old alignment put forth in the previous chapter.

C. Summary

Assuming the best of coverage by NHI and HMO legislation, and the already enacted manpower programs, the migrants would be able to benefit quite a lot, but there would be many gaps that would still have to be covered additionally. Environmental, occupational, and nutritional problems would go completely uncovered, and the basic problem of poverty would be untouched. Although partially ameliorated, problems with mobility, discrimination, and rural medical capacity would be far from completely solved. Special outreach and coordination arrangements to adjust the medical care systems and migrants to each other would be needed, and it would still be very helpful to have a constant monitoring capacity to check on the migrants' health continuously. All those functions, many of which could be served by regional health centers, would be needed in addition to ideal NHI and HMO developments; to the extent those developments were not ideal, even more extra functions would need to be added.

In anticipation of these health policy developments, two basic strategies were offered to the MHP and any other programs that could cooperate. Both alternatives aim at achieving a common end-point of regional health care centers financed basically through NHI, with many costs and services supplied by HMOs, with manpower acquired to a certain extent from the manpower programs, and with basic organization and all the necessary additional services supplied by special migrant money. The "core" strategy would consist of building up as many centers as possible previous to the NHI legislation, but keeping their expansion minimal, with only a "critical mass" present. The intent would be to use NHI money as fast and fully as possible when it should come. The "full scale" strategy would consist of developing to their full potential as many regional health care centers as possible. The idea here would be that as much present services as possible would be produced, and capacity to use NHI money fast and fully would not be much impaired. On the basis of six criteria, the "full scale" strategy appears better overall than the "core" strategy, but in reality these two different strategies are two separate points on a spectrum, and skilled and creative administration could blend them and adapt them to changing national and varied local situations. To carry out any of these projected tasks new personnel in a changed organizational setting are needed.

V CONSEQUENCES OF MIGRANT HEALTH POLITICS ON SUBSTANTIVE POLICY FOR THE MIGRANT HEALTH PROGRAM AND PROJECTS

A. The Necessity for Migrant Input, and Administrative Techniques

The description of the political history and relationships of the MHP make it clear that the organizations composed of and directly representing migrants were never part of the political exchange process. True, there were many parties involved who claimed generally to speak for the migrants' interest. Irrespective of claims, however, it is evident that all parties taking part in the process benefited to a greater or lesser extent. The combination of participation of these groups and absence of participation by migrant-based groups, produced a program with characteristics disadvantageous to the migrants at both project and program level.

If anything, recent health policy events have increased the danger of program dilution from the migrants' point of view. Health advocate groups (e.g., the American Public Health Association) which have supported health care programs for the poor may set a higher priority on their own professional field of health care organization reform than on equalization, and may opt to support the former aspect of NHI rather than the latter in lobbying, or may accept HMO legislation in lieu of strong, equalizing NHI. More directly, administrative officials in HEW and HSMHA, who in the past have sometimes attempted to merge the MHP with the Partnership for Health Program [314(e)] for a tidier comprehensive health package, and for a possibility to shift funds around rather freely, may be atrracted to merge the MHP with general HMO efforts. The HSMHA administrator's order in 1970-71 to the new Migrant Health branch chief to convert all MHP projects to the prepaid principle was the first step in that direction. If impressive migrant projects were to be built up in areas, pressure from the surrounding rural areas to deliver similar benefits to all would encourage efforts to use MHP money to satisfy those demands. Furthermore, there would be no diminution of the traditional pressures on the MHP to satisfy many non-migrant groups.

It is difficult to solve this problem by any other means than finding some way for the migrants to enter into the political exchange process as directly and powerfully as possible, so they can participate in the traditional American political way. Any other solution would necessarily entail someone else's acting in the migrants' behalf without direct responsibility to them. Such an arrangement would violate the basic Madisonian theory of government, and would give no assurance that migrants would be better served than they are today. The major alternative would be to depoliticize the program and give its direction over to an insulated non-partisan board of some sort. But American programs simply do not operate that way. So the question becomes, then, how to effect entry of migrants into the political field of migrant health. (Note that entry of the migrants into the political exchange process involved in the MHP is *not* advocated with the hope that such action will lead to fuller participation of the migrants in political life in general, although that could be one side effect. It is advocated strictly for self-protection in the field of health.)

Involving migrants can be considered at three levels, the local project level, the federal program level, and the congressional and departmental levels.

At the *local project level,* there are four processes the migrants should take part in. First, within the project they should take part in the policy-making process that involves initial planning and implementation and subsequent feedback control operations. Otherwise, the provider group will make policy with their own priorities unavoidably intruding in some areas where they should not. (For examples, refer to Chapter 2 on evaluation of the "classical" MHP.) Second, in interaction between the project and the program the migrants' voice should be strong again. Not only do these interactions often concern the specific operations of the project, and thus deal with matters directly concerning consumers, but programs are often influenced in their external relations to take stands that depend on the attitude of their constituent projects. Examples of such instances should be the program's testimony on a proposed requirement for migrant input in projects, or the program's selection of personnel from the NHSC, or cooperation with other agencies with varying ideologies and behavior patterns.

Third, the migrants should participate in any relationships the project might have with Congress, in testimony on appropriations or changes in the law. Ulterior motives–most often unconscious, probably–on the part of others who testify and influence resulted in program deviations that were injurious in the past. If migrants have ulterior motives in testifying, they will at least be their own, and formulated with their own set of priorities. Existing projects in a congressman's district form a base of power that the congressman is obliged to deal with–in those dealings it is better than the project be dealing with migrant priorities than any others.

Fourth, just as with dealing with the congressman, when a project deals with the local community–the medical providers including doctors and hospitals, local governments, the general populace–it is once again important that it be the migrants' point of view represented. An example: aggressive young physicians or administrators controlling a project might want to fight a war with private medicine for their own reasons, whereas migrants might see it in their interest to compromise and not risk prohibition from service at the local hospital.

If the necessity for migrant participation at the project level is clear, exactly how it should be achieved is not. Rather many different experiments with consumer participation in health and other fields have been tried, but no clear answers have yet emerged.

Two non-mutually exclusive models of project organization seem to be the best bets to ensure migrant participation in each of the four functions. One is the board model, where binding policy is set by a board of directors, whose membership is composed of enough consumer representatives to ensure migrants a strong and predominant voice in the four functions. It is clear from documented experience that little worry needs be spent on problems of protecting the providers in these arrangements, since they are endowed with many natural advantages in any contests for power with the consumers of their services. The providers' social class and sophistication, their ability to go elsewhere with skills the project needs, and their expertise in the substance of medical care convey heavy advantages in any test of strength. These advantages are strengthened if the providers themselves belong to an institution like a medical school or a health department. The project structure, then, must confer advantages to the migrants sufficient to counteract the natural provider advantage. Projects initiated by migrant groups themselves are thus to be preferred, and institutionally sponsored projects with weak migrant participation aspects, such as an advisory committee, to be rejected. In the middle is the area for judgment, with variations in different local situations allowed for.

The second model worth considering is that of industrial democracy, where all workers in the project would cooperate democratically in setting project policy. It would be necessary, then, to hire migrants or at least those from families of farm workers as employees, and to structure decision-making in a manner to offset the natural predominance of the providers. Practice with this form of operation has been extensive in Yugoslavian health centers with apparently satisfactory results.

At the *program level* three separate functions in which it would be desirable to have migrant influence can be identified. These are program-project interaction, program-bureaucracy interaction, and program-Congress interaction. If migrant influence were directly added at this level, different types of project sponsors would be found, more aggressiveness might be produced in dealing with other parts of the bureaucracy that might aid migrants, and the Congress would be given a conduit to hear the migrants' point of view that it had a difficult time getting before.

One way migrants could exercise this influence would be through strong review committees at both central and regional levels dominated by migrants. Objections can be found to this—the difficulty of review committee control, efforts by review committee members to favor their own area (but at least this pressure would benefit a migrant, not an extraneous, group). On the other hand, arming such a group with funds to conduct or have conducted evaluation processes might be quite effective. As at the project level, a second way of obtaining migrant influence would be to employ many migrants as workers and institute cooperative democratic policy-making. At the program level, no current migrants, but only ex-migrants or those related by race and socioeconomic background would be possible, but they might prove to be quite effective. If objections should be raised to such a solution, one should recall the example of regulatory agencies that are regularly staffed by those connected with the industries in question. The usual explanation given is that these people have the requisite expertise. Since the MHP is supposed to *help* migrants rather than regulate them, the case is made *a fortiori.* Since even minority group members in professional, bureaucratic positions are likely to have goals diverging from the consumers of care, it would be unwise to rely solely on the worker influence device to ensure program responsiveness. Whatever the solution, however, it is evident that the migrants should have means to influence events at the program level.

The third level of desired participation of migrants in the political exchange process is the *congressional and departmental level.* Major decisions concerning migrant health are made there with the aid of lobbying interests, although it must be admitted that on the migrant health issue the impact of private lobbying after passage of the initial law seems to have been minimal. The impact of lobbying from the executive branch is always great, however, and constitutes a clear and present danger to migrant health as the issues of medical care develop. Ability to counter this influence is clearly necessary.

To a significant extent migrant participation at the local project and program levels could have the desired effects at the congressional and departmental levels. Local projects could influence their local congressmen, and in addition could testify before and otherwise inform the relevant committees. The departmental level could be influenced by the program, newly reflective of the migrant point of view.

In this case, as in the case of migrant influence on the program albeit to a lesser extent, it would seem problematical to what extent the individual projects would be able to exert influence. A somewhat unorthodox way to aid such influence might be suggested: that the individual projects form an association that would be capable of representing the collective opinions of the projects, as well as providing appropriate reports and such. More concerted and analytic efforts would thus be possible by the usual lobbying means, and would reflect a good deal of migrant opinion, although undoubtedly with a bias born of their commitment to the projects. This idea has already been implemented in the case of the neighborhood health centers.

Of more immediate relevance would be the case of the United Farm Workers. This organization is genuinely migrant-based, has growing prestige and power, and could easily become an influential force at the top levels we are discussing. Certainly their views would represent a biased one, based on their perception of the primacy of organizing, but at least that bias would be a genuinely migrant bias. Furthermore, as was noted earlier, much can be said in favor of viewing union organization, with consequent improvement of the political-economic powerlessness complex, as a primary health objective. Even if their efforts were small, their influence might well serve as a check to other extraneous influences at the top levels.

B. The Technical Possibility of Community Representation

At the three necessary influence levels, then, several techniques seem possible to add the voice of the migrants to the political exchange process. To be able to use these techniques, however, certain prerequisites are necessary. The basic problem is this: how does one obtain a representative voice from the migrants in projects and programs when one of their major problems to begin with is that they have not been able to participate in the traditional political system and develop leadership through that formal organizational means? Associated problems are how does one obtain representation from a mobile population that often does not form a real community in their upstream locations, and how does one deal with the migrants' usual lack of organizational experience, formal organizational skills, and basic educational abilities thought necessary for organizational functioning?

First, the local project level. In trying to implement the board model of migrant participation—that is, where project policy is decided upon by a board which is heavily represented with migrants—it is obviously important to derive membership on the board that is truly representative of the consumer community. First of all, is there a coherent consumer community? In home-base areas, there is a stable consumer community composed of migrants and non-migrants alike. Most live in general residential areas, but some do live in special camps. Although these communities have not been formally described, it seems that there is a spectrum of migrant activity from those families who never migrate, to those who sometimes do, to those who never do. Even among those who always do, there is a period of about six months or more each year when they occupy the same house every year. This applies to all home-base areas. These communities invariably have institutions which may be widely based or particular, loosely- or tightly-knit.

In a great many upstream areas, especially the more important ones, there are two types of communities. One is that of so-called "settled-out migrants," who generally have agriculturally related jobs that are stable enough to enable them to stop or reduce the extent of their migrating. (They are eligible for project services under the present law as "agricultural workers.") Although from the same cultural group as the migrants, these permanent residents are rather better off economically. The second type of community is that of the migrants proper, who generally settle temporarily in camps, most often *not* the same ones year after year. The camps are generally privately owned by growers, and vary in size. The first group, the "settled-out migrants," generally live in the same area and have organizations much as do the home-bases. The migrants in camps apparently do not have organizations, although labor union recruiting does go on there. There are also some migrants who do not live in camps on the road—these are apparently fewer in number than the others, and do not form a community, although they sometimes have contact with the other two groups.

So, given that there generally is a community, how is genuine representation produced for the health center? A good deal of work has been done on this subject by many kinds of community workers, and much experience exists, if not too much with migrant workers. It is generally considered possible to obtain such representation through (1) existing organizations and/or (2) a specifically developed organization for the project in question. The question of how one goes about doing this manipulation without being counter-productive in community development is not at all clear, and constitutes a major dilemma, with many arguments being offered many ways. Basically, it would seem logical that widely-based and consumer-accepted organizations—such as a cooperative, for example, or in some areas the union—could form a parent organization for a project, and develop special mechanisms for it. A more particular organization, with more limited support, might be appropriate for contributing representatives to the controlling board. Under certain conditions this kind of an organization could sponsor a project primarily, if provisions for enlarged representation were made. Finally, community development by special community workers specifically for the purpose of forming a representative organization to sponsor a project would also be possible, although it would take much longer than the above.

In the upstream areas differences between the interests of the "settled-out migrants" and the more widely traveling migrant would be bound to arise, with power lodged more solidly with the former. The fellow-feeling and movement between the two groups, (although movement is predominantly one way), would ameliorate these problems. In addition, it is possible to have direct checks. For one, the camps could elect members to the board on a temporary basis, with obvious problems of continuity for specific planning, organizational relationships on the board, and individual development. For another, qualified "wild-card representatives," specially trained to be a roving representative in the home-base area, could be officially empowered to join the board whenever they turn up on their travels.

As for the problem of ability of migrants to work as board members, this has been shown in various efforts, most notably in health projects in the San Francisco Bay area, to be solvable. The general ability of many members, accumulated experience, and special attention to training for their jobs has proved a successful formula.

Despite all the uncertainties with the board model of project control, and the particular problems migration poses, it does seem warranted to recommend such steps as feasible. In fact, community organization in readiness for health projects would seem an appropriate step to take in anticipation of NHI.

The second model of migrant participation in project control calls for substantial hiring of migrant workers to work in the projects, and democratic control of the projects by the workers. This type of organization has had somewhat less vogue in America than the board-control system, but has had some trials here, and is the basis for organization of local health services in Yugoslavia. The main problems here would appear to be (1) simply instituting an unfamiliar system and (2) ensuring that those employed were genuinely representative of the consumer group. Neither should prevent controlled and serious attempts to institute worker participation from succeeding, although the effort in mounting such efforts would be considerable, and would require creative administration at both program and project levels.

If real migrant participation can be effected at the project level, implementing migrant input at the program level would be considerably facilitated. Just as at the project level, the two leading candidates for means of migrant participation are the representative board system and the workers representation system. Two types of representatives would be appropriate to serve on the board in a capacity representing migrants: representatives of farm worker organizations not directly connected with the MHP and representatives of migrants involved with MHP projects. Neither should be much of a problem recruiting, if local organization of projects worked out properly, although there might be a problem of their being able to act effectively—as indeed there is with many board of non-poor persons. Just as with local project boards, specific short-term training would probably be a helpful step.

As for the worker model, recruitment from socioeconomic backgrounds similar to those of the migrants would present some difficulties initially, but these would tend to decrease over time. Community organization specialists would be relatively easier than medical care organization specialists, but even the latter are now being produced by schools of public health. Furthermore, enough neighborhood health centers have been operating for a long enough time now, so that many minority group members with relevant health experience are available. As the MHP projects develop, they should constitute another source of personnel; in addition, certainly not all of the personnel would have to be representative. In sum, then, both elements of control at the program level should be possible to implement, particularly if efforts at the project level are successful. The departmental and congressional levels would be influenced as migrant representation infiltrated the projects and the program.

C. Summary

In the past the MHP has functioned politically in much the same way as most programs: the supportive forces have received benefits in exchange for their support, and elements that could have been mobilized to block the program were neutralized by recognizing their interests in various ways. Conspicuous by their absence in this exchange process were groups directly representing and composed of migrants. Unless this situation is changed, the MHP will continue to suffer unwonted distortion of policy. In the American context the only real solution is to find a way to deal the migrants into the game.

Just as the non-migrant interests influence three levels, the local project, the program, and the departmental and congressional, so must the migrants be able to influence those levels. At the project level, they must be able to take part in four different functions: planning, implementation, and feedback control; project-program interactions; project-Congress interactions; and project-local community interaction. Two models of organization could accomplish this, the board model and the industrial democracy model. At the program level migrants should have direct influence on the functions of program-project interactions, program-Congress interactions, and program-bureaucracy interactions. A review board with evaluation powers and/or democratic employee control of program policies could effect such migrant influence. At the congressional-departmental level, projects and program are able to be quite influential; therefore, proper implementation of migrant influence at the two lower levels should contribute much to influence at the third level. To facilitate conveyance of the voices of the projects, a special association of the projects might be formed just for that purpose. The largest and most prestigious migrant organization is UFW; their influence at the top levels—as well as elsewhere—would also be desirable.

The major problem with implementing the above suggestions is difficulty in obtaining true and strong representation from migrant communities, with their lack of a tradition of formal representation, mobile populations, and educational and experiential disadvantages. Coherent communities do exist, however, especially when one takes note of interaction between migrant and non-migrant farm workers, and organizational development can be used to develop democratic representation in projects, and thus ultimately at other levels. The lag time intrinsic to such development suggests an additional role for the MHP in anticipation of NHI passage—community development with a health aim. Although stationary farm workers can influence projects in ways consonant with migrant interests for the most part, it is still advisable to have direct migrant representation in projects supplied by camp elections, and appointment and training in home-base areas. Training for board members and general experience should make their performance acceptable. Problems of implementation of employee policy-making would be unfamiliarity with technique and problems of representation, neither of which should prove an insuperable obstacle.

Implementation of the new program level strategies for migrant influence should not be excessively difficult technically, especially if the local projects would develop as suggested.

It can be concluded that introduction of migrant input at all levels of the MHP is necessary and technically possible.

VI POLITICAL POSSIBILITIES OF MAKING THE SUGGESTED MHP CHANGES

This section shall try to use the political factors depicted so far to project the basic initial attitudes of the groups and persons we have found to be involved and important, and try to estimate possibilities for new MHP legislation on that basis.

Three separate changes suggested for the MHP can be defined, and we can see how support and opposition would be lined up regarding each. The first change was suggested by considering alternative technical solutions to the migrant health problem—regional health centers seems the best alternative. The second change was suggested by considering the political interaction and exchange process surrounding the MHP—inclusion of migrant influence in MHP projects seemed to be indicated. The third change, suggested by administrative considerations, was creation of an organizational unit more independent of the influence of the surrounding health bureaucracy, more motivated to seek change, more capable of devising new solutions to migrant health problems, and less oriented to performing routine grants adminstration. An additional administrative change, suggested by this chapter, was that migrant influence be directly introduced at the program level.

A. Change in the Technical Mission of the MHP

It would be easiest to find support for changing the MHP's technical mission. HEW and HSMHA officials would advance their general health policy strategy by adjusting the MHP's mission to accord with it. HEW has been eager to make changes of organization in the health system without significant new expenditures. HSMHA has been anxious to do the same, and wants to be regarded as the home of the HMO effort. In the fall of 1971 the HSMHA administrator even instructed the chief of the Migrant Health Branch to convert as many MHP projects as possible to the HMO type arrangement. The Migrant Health Branch chief tried to comply with this direction by strengthening the already ongoing efforts to eliminate the small-sized MHP projects.

HEW and HSMHA might want to use the MHP as the camel's nose under the tent. Big and conspicuous programs are always closely watched by rival groups—Congress, AMA, hospitals, insurance companies, medical schools, etc. The inclination of HEW to move on its own is thus checked. The MHP, however, is a low-salience program, watched by few and affecting few. HEW can move much more easily in that milieu, and it thus provides a vehicle HEW can use to start trends in motion, unobserved by potential opposition.

The health and migrant subcommittees in Congress are also likely to be supportive. Kennedy's Health Subcommittee will be mainly concerned with the overall health picture. Generally supporters of reorganization, they will look on the technically rational approach to migrant health as a step forward for their views, and one uncomplicated by persistent political battles. The Subcommittee on Migratory Labor will look on the changes as rational for better health care for the migrants and will welcome the added visibility the larger health centers will provide.

Congressman Rogers will tend to be positive toward the change, but with reservations. On the one hand, he has been a supporter of health care reorganization, but cautious to avoid upsetting powerful factions, and is eager to be known as a knowledgeable and progressive leader in health. Furthermore, he would have few worries that his home district would be adversely affected, since he holds quite enough power in Congress to control that. On the other hand, he would be unwilling to incur the displeasure of any comrades in the House if their areas were to lose their current MHP projects. He would also be nervous that new, large centers might cause trouble for local establishments in other counties, which would reflect adversely on him, and jeopardize his other health efforts. Furthermore, Representative Rogers would be suspicious that the new approach would be in reality simply satisfying the wishes of health professionals who wanted to experiment and didn't care too much about service. He would have to be convinced that the change really meant more overall benefit for the migrants. His general belief is that the MHP resources should be spread equally; only strong technical evidence and support from trusted health advisors would induce his support. But, since the case for regional health centers is strong, and since Rogers generally responds to technical reasoning, he would probably support the change. He would be further encouraged by the prospect of making another progressive move in health and its effect on his image, and would be convinced that political opposition would not be great. Although reluctant at first, he would become supportive.

The role of the newly formed Subcommittee on Agricultural Labor in the House would surely be that of support. As with the Senate groups, they would be fairly easily convinced of the desirability of the change and would be risking nothing politically. Their support, however, might not mean much.

The "new" migrant advocate groups would certainly support the change. They would be easily convinced that the old approach was faulty, the new suggested one better; they would have little to lose by the change and a battle victory to be gained.

The American Public Health Association would be another organization quite likely to support the change. They strongly support reorganization of health care along the lines of HMOs, and support health programs for the poor in general. Some of their leaders have been involved in the MHP before and have supported changes such as this one.

Some of the church groups that have supported the MHP in the past are also likely to support the change to big, comprehensive projects, if they are convinced that such a change would really benefit the migrants. These church groups themselves in many instances would derive no less from the MHP if the change were to be made, since they would still participate at the local and national levels.

Finally, the grantees of the new projects funded in 1970 should be strong supporters of the change to make the MHP based entirely on projects like theirs. Such a change would assure the survival and growth of these new projects and possibly provide a constituent base for further efforts in the health field or others. Groups that would expect to be grant recipients if policies were changed would also be possible supporters, including in rare instances projects of the old type that would expect to be upgraded.

The attitudes of local areas would be mixed. As was noted, health departments standing to lose projects would be opposed. They would be joined by some of the local populace who value the protection rendered them by the MHP immunization service and by those who are aware of the plight of the migrants locally and would be reluctant to see them lose the little bit of help they had. Local areas that never had a migrant health grant, but would lose the opportunity of ever getting one by adoption of the new strategy, would never enter into the picture at all, since they would be insensible to the possibilities. Areas with prospects of obtaining a new large-scale project might react favorably if they had an establishment grantee ready to take charge—an example would be one of the few counties with a high-powered and opportunistic health department. Otherwise, there would be no local reaction at first. After projects had been started, local medical societies would tend to be opposed to big projects with competing services and threatening forms of organization, but would find it difficult to fight the projects on that basis, given the growing support for the corporate forms of practice. If the 1970 experience can be used as a guide, the more important determinant of local physicians' reactions will be the question of sponsorship. Depending on sponsorship, the medical societies' attitudes could vary from strong opposition to weak support.

Since the attitudes of local areas would be mixed, so would the attitudes of the congressmen who represent them. The most constant and intense opponents of change would be the health departments, both state and local, who might be losing grants. We have seen that those elements do not have much effect on Congress, however, especially since there are more important local medical influences to be dealt with. Just as the reaction of the medical societies would be expected to come during or after the stage of policy formation, when their local area actually became threatened with a new project, and just as their reactions would vary from strong opposition to weak support, we would expect most of the congressmen to follow their lead. Since there would be relatively few areas affected at first, however, and they would be likely to come up as a series rather than all at once, the effect would be thereby weakened. Furthermore, the fact that health is now a recognized major issue might make the congressmen more cautious with their steps, and make them hesitate to take a stand, lest they be bound to one side of an issue that might become embarrassing.

The second line of communication for the health departments, up through the Public Health Service, has been shown to be much weakened in the last ten years. Still, the health departments would find some support in the regional offices of HEW, where many old line officials are still in charge, and among some few elements of the "classical" MHP still to be found in headquarters. These subordinate HEW forces, however, would not be very powerful in policy making.

The American Medical Association would probably oppose the change to big projects. Such projects would provide competition with local practitioners whereas the old projects did not, and ideological conflicts would be evident as well. Although the AMA would be generally opposed to the corporate form of organization, for the same reason as with local medical societies, the big issue for them would be sponsorship. Several local areas have been "burned" before by the 1970 projects, and the AMA is thus aware of the danger. The chairman of the Rural Health Committee would be likely to sense the threat before the local societies and push the AMA to react accordingly, although a certain lag time would necessarily be present. They would act, however, with recognition that the major issues of NHI and HMOs were still to be fought, and would moderate their approach for that reason. It would seem unlikely that the AMA would decide to "draw the line" at the MHP.

The sum balance of political weight would favor regional health centers for the MHP. If old money were to be withdrawn from traditional projects and reallocated to new ones, much more opposition would be provoked than if only new money were allocated for regional health centers. But since opposition from health departments does not seem all that threatening, reallocation of funds could be included on the agenda, perhaps on a phased basis, sparing the most powerful potential critics until the end. In any event, change in the technical mission of the MHP emerges as a clear possibility.

B. Adoption of Migrant Input at the Project Level

Two different models of administration have been suggested for this proposed change, the board model and the industrial democracy model, each of which could be used alone or in combination with the other. In addition to these alternatives, many degrees of participation are possible, and the issue will be negotiable along these lines. Here, the attitudes of the various parties to the general idea of migrant input must be considered.

Some rather strong and important support for migrant input in project policy making comes from the Senate. The Mondale Amendment to the Migrant Health Act in 1970 tried to assert that migrants should participate fully in project development and continuing decision making. Senator Mondale has been replaced by Senator Stevenson and then Senator Nelson in the chairmanship, and support for this concept has probably weakened somewhat. On the other hand, the replacement of Senator Yarborough by Senator Kennedy as chairman of the Subcommittee on Health has probably strengthened support. Meanwhile, in the House, the newly established Subcommittee on Agricultural Labor would be expected to support migrant input strongly, although with questionable effect.

The "new" migrant advocate groups would be expected to stand foursquare behind migrant input, since this is in accordance with their prevailing ethos. The MHP-projects funded in 1970 can also be expected to support migrant input in the main, since most of them are founded on the same principle themselves. Not only would their ideology and beliefs be involved, but adopting that ideology for the whole program would give the 1970 projects a good deal of protection they do not now enjoy. Establishment of sister projects would give them a better hold on the program in negotiations or other situations where they might need allies.

The American Public Health Association would most likely be supporters here, since those most involved in the migrant issue in the APHA are known to support the idea. Some of the church groups, notably the Migrant Ministry, striving to be modern in their ideology, might also back the idea.

An additional factor would be the movement set in motion by the "change-agents" with the Guidelines and 1970 projects themselves. The official MHP regulations include provisions for a Project Policy Board with at least 51 percent migrant representation. On a more personal basis, the present chief of the Migrant Health Branch has remained committed to the principle of migrant input.

Opposition to migrant participation in the form of a strong policy board could be strenuous. In negotiating over the 1970 amendments Representative Rogers was successful in considerably watering down the thrust of the Mondale Amendment. Rogers stressed that the whole community should be involved, not just the migrants, and that considerable latitude should be given to the project administrators. He is always very sensitive to the position of the establishment community and would be most unlikely to risk their displeasure even if he were convinced that migrant participation were a good thing. Migrant input could be viewed by him as a threat to the whole constituency he will rely on for his larger area health moves.

Congressman Rogers is far from unique in Congress with his doubts about consumer input. From OEO experiences in non-health community action projects, "consumer participation" is viewed as troublesome without compensatory benefits. Thus, the atmosphere of the Congress will be against migrant input, at least if seen in that light.

The HEW and HSMHA Administration as presently constituted would also be counted among the opponents of strong migrant participation. HEW's general policy on consumer participation is at best a cautious one. The HSMHA administrator has been heard on more than one occasion to voice his strong opposition to any actions of the MHP that would upset the local community and to consumer participation aspects of the 1970 new projects in particular. In both cases the current establishment in the local areas is counted as the major constituency and strong consumer participation is correctly seen as a method to cut others into that power. The lower level, traditional part of the PHS in most regional offices would be very wary of migrant input as an unneeded obstacle to dealing between professionals and government agencies. Like the Migrant Health Branch chief, however, many of these lower level attitudes have softened considerably over the past few years, and some regions speak quite directly of the need for migrant input.

The American Medical Association would be quite negative, as would the state and local health departments, since they would also see the change as a shift of power from their hands to those of others. Local governments would also generally oppose the changes on the basis that the projects would then be acting to set up alternative centers of power in the local communities, but these units of government would be expected to act only after the fact, not in anticipation. Local medical societies would be strongly opposed, of course, although once again such opposition would manifest itself only after establishment of a local threat. The local congressmen would respond to all these pressures by being negative to substantial migrant input, or at least stressing the need for professional input as well.

Also standing ready to moderate any strong migrant participation moves would be large institutions, such as universities, that would expect to mount a migrant project.

Some of the more traditional church groups could be rather opposed to migrant participation, on the general grounds of their directive philosophy as well as the specific grounds that they might be concerned with starting projects themselves and would not want to be overly burdened.

Different motivations among these potential opponents of substantial migrant input can be discerned. A general distrust of "consumer participation" would be one level; a deeper level would be opposition to a redistribution of power in local communities. More specifically, medical and health groups might be opposed to redistribution of influence in the medical area.

Various steps could be taken to neutralize some of this opposition. One important step would be to avoid the rhetoric of consumer participation, which will often prove to be only inflammatory. Instead, it would be well to concentrate on the essentials behind the words, which may not be so threatening: adjustment of services to ongoing demand, employment of low-income minority groups, cooperation in decision-making, etc. It would also be well to avoid making the goal seem to be change in the power relations of the whole community, but rather just concentrate on the projects themselves. Emphasizing the natural advantage of professionals in steering projects might make it seem less threatening to have migrants represented in apparently strong numbers—the fact is that even middle-class consumers in cooperative medical plans almost always have surrendered leadership to physicians and other professionals.[7] The training and nurturing that migrant representatives would receive should be offered with the explanation that they need such to be responsible and to fulfill their roles properly. Other steps softening the approach could probably also be developed.

In fact, however, all opposition cannot be neutralized, because there *is* an influence realignment to be made. The local medical providers will have interests sometimes opposed to the migrants' interests; likewise with universities if they were to become involved with the MHP. But the days when these groups could have their way exclusively are clearly over, and they know it. In addition to the supportive groups mentioned, other factors give strength to the move toward migrant input. Generally, consumer input is an accepted concept, even if the means of management is not. Furthermore, beyond the governmental motivations we have mentioned above, it is in the federal government's interests to have a balance of forces in projects and programs; if there were not to be such a balance the government would have surrendered its power of control to whichever agent it was that overcame the balance. As an organization, the government would not like to lose its power to private medicine, a large organization such as a medical school or a hospital, or to migrant workers. As a political body, HEW would like to please Senate, House, and all the other parties with influence; giving each a small share of the action could satisfy each party politically, and keep HEW in control, satisfying their own organizational demand. Finally, the fact that current MHP regulations include migrant input gives the important advantage of precedent to advocates of that approach.

Despite these strengths, compromises might well have to be made. Even if special factors would ensure adoption of strong migrant input in MHP projects, opponents could scuttle all program change in retaliation. Less important than the specific regulations and specific numbers of migrants on the board would be the basic situation of a new MHP project, staffed by professionals recruited for that specific project and thus for the most part sympathetic to migrant input ideas, giving a good basic working situation amenable to migrant input.

Probably the biggest threat to migrant input would not be variations in the representation formula for boards, etc., but rather a project administrator controlled by an organization other than the project itself. Even if the board would be mixed and ineffective, and the administrator rather independent, if the project were not under the umbrella of a large and powerful organization, the administrator would pursue the goals dictated by forces around the project. If, on the other hand, the project were part of a university or hospital complex, even a strong board would have difficulty restraining the administrator from identifying with the parent organization and making moves calculated to increase his standing in that organization, along with direct interference in project operations by the parent institution. An independently located project would clearly be an asset to the migrants and would be a very realistic possibility, for with the diversity of interests involved in the issue, no one would like to see the MHP caught up in one of the other's institution.

Although the forces supporting migrant input into MHP projects are strong, there is significant opposition. Three types of motivations stand behind the opposition: fear of "consumer participation" type activity, opposition to community power redistribution, and opposition to medical care power redistribution. The first two of these motivations can probably be discharged with adjustments of rhetoric and intent. Those forces opposing migrant input because of the third motivation could probably be overcome by the proponent forces, but compromise would be possible and beneficial to the migrants. The greatest danger to the migrants would be incorporation of the MHP projects into larger organizations at the local level, but probabilities favor their independence.

C. Administrative Reorganization of the MHP

The third important suggested change includes: (1) adjusting the administrative arrangements according to Chapter 4; (2) employing many more workers in the MHP who have socio-ethnic ties to the migrant groups; and (3) establishing a review committee composed largely of representatives of migrant groups and migrant participation projects.

The relevant Senate subcommittee would tend to support all three aspects of reorganization although support for the first might be half-hearted. Any increased prominence given to the migrant issue within the bureaucracy would be welcomed and would reflect well in the eyes of their generally liberal constituency. The Health Subcommittee would be concerned, however, that nothing be done to jeopardize their efforts on the broader fronts. Reassignment of capable personnel to the MHP might not be fully supported then. The review committee and ethnic employment issues would also probably be viewed favorably by the Senate because of their generally pro-consumer involvement attitude.

The "new" migrant advocate groups would be fully behind all three proposals, in all likelihood. Their ideology would be consonant with the new approaches and they themselves would be likely to receive increased influence. The 1970 new MHP projects would be counted among the supporters for much the same reasons.

The progressive leadership in APHA would look positively on increased prominence given to a health program for the poor, but would be hesitant to see good people moved into the MHP from other programs. On the other hand, they would form the creation of existing new jobs for their members. This progressive leadership, buttressed by some leaders with special recent experience with the MHP, would also favor migrant involvement in administration and in a review board.

The church groups would tend to favor the new measures, particularly if they were assured that they would have a representative on the review committee. They are striving to be modern in their advocacy beliefs.

HEW would not want to make aggressive moves that might compromise their HMO efforts, and other program initiatives. Chapter 4's suggestions would not, therefore, be popular with them. They would accept the review committee idea, probably, even including a majority of migrant representatives, as an interesting and low-risk experiment in methods of consumer representation. On the other hand, any real power for the committee would be opposed as putting unwanted constraints on HEW's ability to maneuver. The employment of more Chicanos and blacks with agricultural and rural backgrounds as HEW workers would be supported in name, at least. The lower levels of HEW would feel much the same as the higher levels.

The AMA's opposition to MHP changes would center more on the mission change and the migrant input suggestions rather than any reorganization changes. A review committee should be composed substantially of professionals, the AMA would assert. They would not object to employment of minority group members in the MHP administration, providing they were "qualified."

The state and local health departments would view reorganization of the MHP as a threat to their current projects and future prospects and would therefore oppose a change in personnel. A review committee, they would assert, should be composed of persons like those who served in the past. They, too, would not object to employment of minority group members in the MHP administration, providing they were "qualified."

Finally, the opinion of Paul Rogers in the House would be the key. On the one hand, it would appeal to Rogers to give prominence to the MHP effort as a medical care organization issue (in itself increasing his prestige) that might help get HMOs and other reorganization of medical care efforts moving (further increasing his prestige). In addition, he would not mind the prominence given efforts for the poor group that he is most closely associated with, since it would help his standing with liberal sectors. But he would be loath to let the MHP jeopardize chances with the real big issues, NHI and HMOs, and would therefore not want to push much with new organizational efforts.

Rogers would want any review board to have many professional representatives on it, and perhaps relatively few migrants, but otherwise he would be in favor of a review body. This would not be a very strong issue with him. Nor would that of minority employment, which he would accept.

In summary, the reorganization proposals would have some support from the groups concerned only with migrants, but most MHP supporters have bigger stakes in HMOs, NHI, and even other service programs, and would thus not be supportive. Acceptance of focusing prime attention temporarily on migrants would only come if by chance these other efforts stalled at the same time the MHP got a big boost. Almost all groups would approve a review committee, but the composition and powers of the committee would be at issue. Possibilities here would be chancy and subject to compromising. Employment of persons associated socio-ethnically with the migrant population as officials in the MHP would be unopposed in theory. In practice, it would be up to the migrant advocates to produce the proper candidates and support them. The political ingredients for a successful MHP reorganization seem to be present, but luck and a good political cook to mix the ingredients would be required.

D. Summary

Before summarizing the political chances for MHP change, it should be observed that even after passage of NHI legislation and possible subsequent attacks on the existence of the MHP on the grounds of redundancy of effort, the chances of MHP survival are high. The MHP has the force of inertia on its side, a strong set of supporters even in the changing milieu, and virtually no out and out opponents. NHI would even in a sense strengthen the MHP and its ability to attract supporters, since much of the funds would be freed up by replacement by NHI funds, and could then be distributed for organizational and supportive activities, as outlined above, to many more projects. The theoretical framework has also been stated here for the programmatic desirability of retention of the MHP. So, the MHP would be likely to stay.

Enactment of all three suggested changes would appear to be technically feasible, if not certain. Potential support for change in the technical mission of the MHP would appear strong, tied as it would be to the general issue of the reorganization of health care. This change, indeed, is happening even now. The second suggested change, introduction of substantial migrant input at the project level, could be the subject of controversy, although it has made good progress up until now. Concentration on the detailed functions involved, deemphasis of contentious catchwords, and adoption of flexible and innovative administrative techniques could further promote agreement on policies conducive to acceptable migrant input. The third suggested change, administrative reorganization of the MHP, would also seem to be supportable in its three aspects, although much less certainly than the first two. Some good luck, persistent advocacy, and resourceful tactics would be necessary.

VII CLARIFICATION OF TWO IMPINGING ISSUES: THE UNION AND RURAL HEALTH

Two issues have been touched on before, but have not been properly considered in their political context. The first issue concerns the implications of the MHP and the United Farm Workers union for each other; the second issue concerns the connection of the MHP with the more general issue of rural health.

A. The United Farm Workers Union

Two basic observations should be made at the start. First, the UFW represents a traditional American effort to solve the problems of employees in an industry; unionization is a reasonably successful and generally accepted mode of action in such circumstances. Government efforts to aid the population in question directly, on the other hand, is untraditional in the American experience, and has proved generally unsuccessful in the areas it has been tried. The implication, then, is that in interactions between them, the MHP should be deferential to the UFW, and make sure that MHP efforts do not compromise the ultimately more promising efforts of the UFW.

The second observation is that the union issue is very hot politically, and forces very influential with the government strenuously oppose unionization of the farm workers. Severe limitations are thus placed on the MHP in its interactions with the UFW.

The UFW has set about providing for the health of its workers in several ways, as it is traditional for unions to do. In the non-medical care area, they have included pesticide control regulations in the contracts they have negotiated so far, and have prospects for regulation of other occupational and environmental hazards. Additionally, the union's concern with wage rates and employment practices have implications for the prime problem of poverty and through that to health; the very existence of the union has importance for the primal problem of political-economic powerlessness. In all these important health related areas, union action has a great potential.

The UFW has also directly provided medical care services for several years under the Robert F. Kennedy Plan. This plan is supported by employer contribution and union funds, provides limited coverage, and employs physicians at non-competitive wages.

In both medical and non-medical aspects competition between UFW and the MHP can arise. The benefits of unionization are important weapons in the union's organizing efforts; to the extent the government provides those benefits, the organizers' task is perhaps made more difficult. With non-medical health services competition is unlikely, since most of the services are intangible and thus not potent attractions for prospective members, and the government has had no success with these problems for years anyway. The new regional health centers would probably provide no real competition for the potential of contractual agreements by supplying non-medical services. In fact, an attractive model of cooperation would be suggested by the MHP's and UFW's differential abilities: the MHP supplying professional input, such as field surveys, epidemiological work, etc., and the UFW supplying the policy input in their contractual negotiations.

Competition in medical care provision is more likely. That this has not happened so far is due to three factors. An initial lack of serious effort on both sides was the first factor. In the 1960s the UFW was not yet offering medical services to a large extent, and the MHP services were not of sufficient comprehensiveness and excellence that they would make it appear union effort was unnecessary. The second factor was that as both groups started to make serious efforts to provide attractive medical care in the early 1970s, they chose different localities in which to do it. Finally, the third factor is that on the West Coast, at least, the MHP sponsors of new projects are not viewed as inimical to the union. The possible transiency of these factors is patent.

The important question is, if the MHP should in some instances embarrass the UFW by installing a large and excellent medical care center in an area where the UFW has been able to manage only a little bit, how destructive would that be of the union? It would be ironic, indeed, if efforts to provide for the health of the migrants should wind up working against their better interests by impeding unionization. In fact, however, medical services is only one of a panoply of benefits the union has to offer, and although they might be temporarily embarrassed, it is hard to picture a governmental medical care program significantly interfering with the organizing efforts of UFW. If the medical care programs on the local level were organized with provision for migrant input as suggested, the union could simply drop its own efforts (saving the money for other programs) and assert its influence on the MHP center. The total effect might not be so different from what would happen in a directly UFW-run center. In addition, the combination of government sponsorship and union control would relieve the UFW of having to consider the relationship of their centers to more general problems of rural health. In other words, although there is more potential for competition in the medical than the non-medical area, the same possibility for cooperation obtains, and by astute tactics the UFW could turn a potential embarrassment into a distinct asset.

If the MHP project were to have little or no provision for migrant input, a more conflictual situation would develop, to the advantage of no one, most likely. The obnoxious aspects of the health center that would be bound to develop could be exploited by the union in their propaganda, and popular efforts mounted to influence the center from outside rather than inside, thus polarizing the situation. The union would be but little hurt, then, and the health center would find it much rougher. In sum, then, it might be that the MHP cannot hurt the union, but the union can hurt the MHP. If this is so, fears on behalf of the union are groundless, but the MHP should take pains to include the union at the local level just to protect itself.

From the MHP's point of view, a strong argument has been advanced in this study for involving migrants at several programmatic levels, basically through organizations of the farm worker community. For that policy to be carried out the UFW must clearly be represented, since it is the most widespread and vigorous organization among farm workers, although there is no reason for it to monopolize farm worker representation, since other farm worker organizations do exist and should be represented. If the UFW voice were to be missing, the chance for the MHP to receive strong and stimulating migrant input would be diminished.

We are speaking, then, of trying to get strong but balanced representation from within the farm worker community. Wherever the union appears, however, the political opponents of farm worker unionization from *outside* the community will claim a right to be represented. Their claim will be that the MHP is a government program, and as such must be neutral in such issues as unionization. These forces will want the UFW to go unrepresented, or at least be balanced by grower and other local community representation.

From a logical point of view, these claims would be confused ones. Put another way, their assertion would be that the MHP might have implications for others than just migrants and farm workers—as indeed it does—and that everyone thus affected should be represented. This seemingly reasonable point of view has the defect that it is not followed in other programs. Thus, in the Department of Agriculture programs designed to aid farming, there is no representation from farm workers, although they are clearly affected by policies connected with harvesting. To have overall community representation in the program designed to help the farm worker specifically, and to lack that overall representation in the programs designed to help everyone, would clearly constitute treating the farm workers differently from others, and iniquitously.

In point of political fact, however, claims advanced by the growers, medical societies, and other groups are bound to find a great deal of support in the government by the routes previously described. But, despite the obvious power of the anti-union forces, the issue of health centers is hardly central for them, and certainly at the beginning of the new efforts their claims would not be pressed hard. Most probably, union representation could be included as part of representation of the migrant community without the spurious "balancing" forces, and defended later under any attack by the argument put forth above. Certainly, the union would be more than happy to exchange anti-union representation on the MHP for union representation of the Department of Agriculture and Department of Labor programs.

Another approach would also be possible. If MHP grants go to groups that are fairly firmly based on the farm worker population, such as some of the 1970 project groups, informal influence of the union groups might be all that would be necessary for proper coordination, and the possibility of confrontation with the anti-union groups avoided. Such an arrangement might be preferable to the union, since it would avoid diluting their organizing efforts. In any event, it would appear that the specter of anti-union power would be less than it would appear on first inspection.

To sum up: the MHP might cause some competition for the UFW, but that would probably turn out to be rather unimportant from the UFW's point of view, so the MHP would probably not have to be too careful about the possibility of impeding the more important UFW. On the other hand, the UFW's cooperation in some form would be necessary for the MHP to have proper farm worker input and make the MHP a success. Although the opposition to the union is influential, the MHP would be a low salience item for them, and opposition to the UFW cooperation would come late, if at all. Several avenues of action would then be possible, but it is likely that the UFW input could be maintained and a representative farm worker point of view perpetuated.

B. The Rural Health Issue

Many of the problems of the non-migrating agricultural workers, the rural poor, and even the rural non-poor, coincide. The implications of a program to serve just one part, albeit the most needy part, of this larger group should now be considered.

With a shortage of services in rural areas, there is bound to be competition for use of these services. To the extent that migrant workers use local resources, they take them away from others in the community. If special resources are brought in to serve the migrants, the others in the community will wonder why only the migrants are served in this way. Both alternatives will lead to resentment from the local permanent community. Since that community has more power than the migrants, it is unlikely that the migrant services will remain superior to those of the rest of the community. (In a two-class system of medical care, it is unlikely that the group with less political-economic power will enjoy superior services.) So, either the services for the rest of the community will get better, or the migrant services will get worse, or both. One of the most likely solutions would be for the migrant centers to be opened up for care for all, which indeed they already are in many instances. If no more money is added into the system, then the result is a dilution of good quality services down to a minimum again, or payment from MHP funds for the care of others, shortchanging the migrants. If more money is added into the system, either through partial payment schemes or governmental payments, then expansion of the services is made possible. (It was in anticipation of this development with NHI that the "full scale" strategy was espoused above.)

What has happened in this hypothetical chain of events is clearly evolution of a migrant health program into a rural health program. Nice as it might be for the communities involved, the fact remains that the MHP winds up diluting its resources for the benefit of non-migrants once again. And we could have followed the chain further to suppose that other communities that do not host migrants wonder why they, with their problems, should be left out of the program, which would lead to spending some money in those communities as well (or at least the ones with powerful congressmen).

The ultimate conclusion is that it is artificial to separate rural residents into different categories, since all partake of the same problems and the same basic solutions. Would it be wise, then, to adopt a strategy of proposing a rural health program? Politically, this would seem to be a poor choice at the moment. Whereas the popular MHP is viewed as an *additive* program, rather than as a *competing* one, a rural health program would be clearly seen as one which sought to redistribute resources to rural areas and away from other areas, such as suburbs. Most probably, the weak redistributive measures already passed by Congress (the manpower programs) are the most that can be passed at the present time. Moreover, the same forces that would be active in pushing the MHP toward rural health contributions (most of the forces we have mentioned before, including health care professionals) would be in a much more powerful position with a rural health program, and it is thus not at all clear that the migrants would benefit, even if a great deal more resources were pumped into the area.

From the migrants' point of view, then, it would be most helpful to keep the MHP population range as it is, open up the centers to others in the community on a graduated fee schedule basis, and try to counter the greater power of others in the community by implementation of the migrant input plans advanced in this report. The fact that the rural health problem is really so deeply intertwined with the migrant health problem that the MHP must inevitably benefit others in rural areas besides the migrants, must simply be accepted, with the realization that many effects are externalities that do not lessen the migrants' benefit.

VIII SUMMARY OF CHAPTER 5

I. Congressional Structure and the MHP

The MHP finds itself mainly in the health policy area in both Congress and the Executive Branch. Specific subcommittees do exist in both House and Senate to deal with migrant-related legislation, and act as internal lobbying units. In the House, however, the Subcommittee on Migrant Labor has little to do with the Subcommittee on Health and the Environment. In general, the MHP is better integrated with health programs than it is with other programs affecting migrants.

II. The Political Forces in Migrant Health

A. From the MHP's beginning, the political communications and exchange system operated to include many interested groups, but not the migrants, who had no effective lobbying group directly responsible to them. The groups who did participate, and thus received benefits, included the following: local medical care providers, local communities in general, growers, state and local health departments, church groups and public spirited citizens, the APHA, and federal officials. Many program decisions that seemed inexplicable from the health administration standpoint are explainable from this political standpoint.

B. In the years following the MHP's establishment, both the general political atmosphere and the specific forces impinging on the MHP have changed. Several local organizations of farm workers have been established. Many new, relatively non-paternalistic migrant advocacy groups have founded. The APHA and the federal government have become more aggressive in medical care experimentation. The AMA has softened its stand against new organized forms of practice. Health departments have a weaker connection with the federal government. HEW is more conservative, but is firmly committed to involvement in financing and organization of health care, and favorable to Chicano interests. The central House figure in health and the MHP is Representative Paul Rogers, who has ambitions to be considered a "health statesman," which ties him in general to health establishment opinion. Ted Kennedy is now chairman of the Senate Subcommittee on Health. He seeks to retain his national liberal constituency, and Chicanos are a pet issue for him. The MHP has remained a generally "popular" program in the Congress.

C. The case of the 1970 new projects reveals some of the political dynamics surrounding the MHP. The most consistent and powerful opposition to the new projects came from local physicians, who seemed to object more to community group sponsorship than to innovative organizations. They objected through the AMA to the federal administration, and through the local congressman, who was usually sympathetic. Support for the new projects came mainly from young liberals in the federal government. HEW got conflicting signals, but gave tacit support to HSMHA to quiet the MHP down. The major influences at the HSMHA level were probably the conservative beliefs of the HSMHA administrator in regard to local project sponsorship, a general unwillingness to incur political opposition, and a specific desire to stockpile medical-political good will for major programs.

III. Health Care Policy Trends

The three major problems from the public's point of view contributing to the current "health crisis" may be described as individual and social cost, equality, and appropriateness of care. The three strongest currents of governmental response are National Health Insurance, manpower programs, and reorganization through Health Maintenance Organizations. Although there are wide options in all the programs, NHI hits mainly at equality, HMOs at cost control and appropriateness, and manpower programs act as a prerequisite for the other two. The manpower programs, already passed, are relatively uncontroversial. HMOs are moderately controversial, most opposition coming from the private physician sector and from those who fear that focusing on HMOs obscures the issue of equality. NHI is highly controversial and highlights a basic internal conflict in the American value system, pitting the value of equality against that of financial equity, and involving very significant transfers.

IV. Consequences of Health Care Policy for Migrants and the MHP

A. Assuming ideal coverage from NHI and HMO legislation, and the manpower programs already passed, the effect on migrant health problems would have the following profile:

poverty	*mobility*	*discrimination*	*rural medical capacity*	*environment*	*occupation*	*nutrition*
0	++	++	++	0	0	0

medical care	*type of care*	*efficiency*	*spillover*
+++	+++	++++	0

Still needed would be the following: a poverty antidote; accessibility provisions, such as special information and registration efforts; direct efforts to supply a sense of community to those who migrate, including regulation of labor practices to minimize travel; antidiscrimination efforts to improve housing, working conditions, etc.; strong manpower and resource redistribution measures; environmental measures; occupational measures; nutrition measures; and an overall surveillance capacity for continued feedback on the state of migrant health. The MHP could improve the scores in many of the above categories if regional health centers were established.

B. Two basic general strategies are suggested for the MHP to follow in anticipation of those health care centers financed basically through NHI, with many costs and services supplied by HMOs, with manpower to a certain extent from the manpower programs, and with basic organization and all the necessary additional services supplied by special migrant money. The "core" strategy would consist of building up as many centers as possible previous to NHI passage, but keeping their size at only "critical mass" levels; the "full scale" strategy would consist of developing to their full potential as many regional health care centers as possible. On the basis of six criteria, the "full scale" strategy appears better than the "core" strategy, but in reality the two strategies are but two points on a spectrum, and skilled administration could blend and adapt them to changing national and varied local situations. To carry out any of these projected tasks new personnel in a changed organizational setting are needed.

V. Consequences of Migrant Health Politics on Substantive Policy for the MHP and its projects

A. Both past and present events indicate that the MHP needs migrant input, and this is supported by the basic Madisonian theory of government. At the local project level, migrants should influence four functions: project operations policy-making, project-program interaction, project-Congress interaction, and project-local community interaction. Two administrative methods are suggested to effect this input: the board model and the industrial democracy model. At the program level, migrants should influence three functions: program-project interaction, program-Congress interaction, and program-bureaucracy interaction. Two suggested administrative methods to effect this are establishment of a review board and industrial democracy. Migrant influence is also desirable at the congressional-departmental level. If migrant input obtains at the project and program levels, it will be reflected at this higher level. In addition, the projects with migrant input could form a voluntary organization to represent their views. Finally, it would be desirable for already existing migrant organizations, the largest being the United Farm Workers, to represent the migrants' interests at the top levels

B. The viability of the above suggestions rests on the possibility of obtaining true community representation. Coherent communities of migrants exist in the home-base areas, and organizations already exist in these communities that can form the basis of representation. In the upstream areas, communities of "settled-out" migrants exist; in addition, most migrants upstream live in camps from which representation can be obtained. An additional form of representation for migrants would be the "wild-card" representative, empowered and trained to represent migrants in the upstream areas. For participation in the board model of migrant input, training and experience have been shown to be effective. At the program level, representation would be fairly easily obtained both from farm worker organizations connected to the MHP and those unconnected to the MHP. Effecting the industrial democracy model at the program level would be facilitated by the increasing availability of minority group professionals, but their independence would be curtailed by bureaucratic limits.

VI. Political Possibilities of Making the Necessary MHP Changes

The major MHP changes suggested in this report can be tested against the political factors laid out in this chapter to assess their feasibility; the political improvement in the MHP's situation over the years is encouraging. Chances for continuation of the MHP despite passage of NHI are high. Support for change in the technical mission of the MHP (to guilding regional health centers) would have a good deal of strength, even if "old money" were to be reprogrammed. Support for adoption of migrant input at the project level would be more problematic, but most opponents could be mollified by tactical alterations, and compromises acceptable to the migrant forces as well as the others could be found. The suggestions for administrative reorganization encompass those made in Chapter 4, plus two made in this chapter, that workers with socio-ethnic ties to the migrants be employed to work at the program level, and that a review committee consisting largely of migrant representatives be established. These recommendations would be feasible, but more difficult to effect than the others.

VII. Clarification of Two Impinging Issues: the Union and Rural Health

A. The MHP would be unlikely to damage organizing efforts of the UFW, but UFW input into the MHP could be very important to achieve the MHP goals. Despite the political opposition to the UFW, such input would be possible if the UFW were willing.

B. Although there are inevitable connections between the MHP and the overall problem of rural health, and although the MHP will surely find itself contributing to the solution of that problem sometimes to the detriment of the migrant, and although a rural health program might have something to contribute to the solution of migrant health, in the near future a large program to improve rural health would seem politically infeasible, and of debatable use to the migrant in any event.

Epilogue

I returned from Sweden in late summer, 1972, armed with a two-inch thick draft of this book. Since the current MHP legislation was due to run out on June 30, 1973, an effort at renewal was imminent. I decided to see if the findings of the study could influence the thinking of the Congress not by publishing it, but rather by presenting it privately. I therefore contacted Jim Mongan of the Senate Finance Committee staff, a friend and former "two-year" man in the Denver regional office of CHS with migrant experience. Jim got me in contact with Brian Biles, a young physician who served as legislative assistant to Democrat William Roy of Topeka, Kansas, a physician-lawyer on the House Subcommittee on Public Health and the Environment.

Faced with a large burden of legislative duties and wishing to serve competently, the subcommittee was in the habit of working cooperatively among members and among staff. At this particular time, fourteen separate authorities were up for renewal and the staff was especially hard pressed. Since I came to Biles well recommended, with an impressively large document presenting a persuasive argument, and we were compatible, and since the MHP could otherwise receive only peripheral attention from the subcommittee, he was happy to work with me. For my part, I was happy to work with someone as enthusiastic and capable as Biles, and happy to work first with the House, since that branch was the more common critical step for liberalizing the MHP.

Working together, Biles and I produced a draft bill (See Appendix F) modeled on the Health Maintenance Organization legislation that Biles had had a large hand in drafting. To the HMO definition of comprehensiveness were added environmental components. To ensure large-sized centers, we first tried to put a minimum price tag of $1 million on each project; in a later draft we tried instead to mandate a minimum of five doctors per center and set a maximum grant at $2-1/2 million, hoping with the latter that the common phenomenon of "the ceiling becoming the floor" would occur—that is, projects would take a maximum figure as a goal to work toward and administrators would feel comfortable with grants about that size. We defined the system by requiring that comprehensive centers be established in "migrant-impacted areas," where 8,000 migrants lived for six or more months of the year, and allowing the centers to serve everyone in that area. (This requirement would define at least twenty-one counties as "high impact.") The upstream projects would be for follow-up of chronic care, coordinating the migrants with services available in the area, and delivering emergency services. Only 15 percent of funds would be available for the in-stream projects.

We tried to ensure consumer input by defining the Project Policy Board membership and functions as had been done in the regulations and by establishing a consumer dominated advisory board for each of the three streams. We called for increased funding to the $50 million level as our best guess of what the House would accept and added provisions for planning and construction grants as in the HMO bill.

I could find no way to attack the problem of administrative reorganization directly. I was too embarrassed even to suggest setting up a separate commission for the MHP, and resolved simply to hope that if the MHP got a big boost in funding and other programs in the CHS were quiescent, there would be a natural flow of energy and expertise to the MHP.

Steve Lawton, counsel to the Subcommittee, liked the draft and the idea of concentrating on high-impact areas was supported by the director of the Palm Beach County Health Department, with whom Lawton was instructed to check. Lawton urged me to coordinate our views with the Ad Hoc Committee to Save the Migrant Health Act and the American Public Health Association. We also wanted to check with the CHS administration. The Ad Hoc Committee was organized by the East Coast Migrant Health Project, the same project led by Catholic Sisters that had been funded in 1970 as a concession to Helen Johnston, the former Migrant Health Branch chief. Interested mainly in renewing the legislation with an increased funding level, their representative was reluctantly persuaded to accept our view of high impact concentration of funds. The APHA agreed with our views, but felt some duty to protect the interests of the in-stream projects, many of them run by APHA constitutents. We agreed on inserting a provision in the legislation to phase in the concentration of funds more gradually. The CHS officials supported our concepts but suggested that they could be implemented on an administrative basis with flexibility of laws retained (although evidence was to the contrary).

The spring of 1973 saw pitched battle between the Administration and the Congress. Of the fourteen health bills at issue, the Administration wanted to terminate the independent authority of ten. They had already resorted to large scale impounding of funds, and writing of regulations to subvert the intentions of the lawmakers. The subcommittee's response was to group the pieces of legislation into several bills with multiple titles, for the sake of both expeditiousness and rationality in considering them. The MHP was placed in the Health Revenue Sharing and Health Services bill, with the other health services programs, Community Mental Health Centers, Community Health Centers, Family Planning, Developmental Disability. Under Administration prodding, the Republicans on the subcommittee continued delaying tactics, and at the end of June, all the old bills were given one year extensions, with the intention of returning to them the following year.

H.R. 11511, the Health Revenue Sharing and Health Services Bill, was introduced to the House on November 15, 1973. The MHP provisions differed from our original draft, but the idea remained constant. H.R. 11511 called for comprehensive projects in high impact migrant areas (6,000 for at least six months of the year, thereby encompassing more than forty counties), but no minimum size for the projects was explicit, and the provision for unitary administration of the center that we had borrowed from the HMO legislation was deleted. The functions of the in-stream projects were widened and made more vague, but after a short phase-in period, only 15 percent of funds were to be allocated there. The consumer input provisions for project governing boards were retained, but the provisions for a program advisory board were dropped. Our suggested funding level was retained, but the provisions for planning and construction were deleted. Finally, in an addition of his own devising, stimulated by his numerous site visits to migrant areas, Rogers inserted a subsection calling for contracts to enforce environmental health standards and to study that problem further. Not more than 10 percent of funds were to be expended on that subsection.

Interestingly, as a consequence of their close proximity in 11511, the provisions for the community health centers legislation were made much like those for the migrant health centers.

Hearings on the bill were held in February 1974. The Administration still pressed its former position that most of the independent authorities should be terminated and that administrative discretion should be relied upon. By this time, however, the impoundment issue had been decisively resolved in favor of the Congress by the courts, and Watergate had dampened the resolve of the GOP sufficiently that Congress was clearly in the driver's seat.

Administration witnesses supported the general thrust of 11511, even down to the details of describing what a migrant health center should do. But they called for administrative flexibility in requiring that specific services be offered by a center and warned that the proposed concentration of funds in high-impact areas would lead to closing some in-stream projects.

Rogers, however, was explicit about his decision to write more detailed bills. He questioned the Administration on the Community Mental Health Centers:

> Mr. Rogers Thank you. Mr. Secretary, what were the HEW proposals that went to OMB on these programs? Did you include any

proposals for new starts, for construction, for financial distress, for community mental health centers which have reached their eight years? Did the Department submit these programs and proposals to OMB?

Dr. Edwards (*Assistant Secretary for Health, HEW*) We did submit our recommendations on these health service programs to OMB. There were some modifications.

Mr. Rogers Some of which were programmatic, were they not, and not just money?

Dr. Edwards Yes, I suspect that you would say programmatic.

Mr. Rogers Which causes me great distress, Mr. Secretary, that the OMB is again into writing programs for health rather than getting to money figures. We have been through this before. I guess we are going to have to start it all over again.

I think we are over the impoundment in the health field. I see the attention there has gone elsewhere for impoundment so I hope we don't have to go into that argument. So, we will address ourselves this year to get them out of writing the health programs. We got them out of withholding the funds so maybe we can get them out of writing the health programs which you ladies and gentlemen ought to be doing because you know a little more about it.

Later in the hearings, in finishing the discussion on migrants:

Dr. Edwards Mr. Chairman, I don't think it is a matter of our disagreeing with anything you wish to accomplish in your Bill but we think there is need for more administrative discretion than you.

Mr. Rogers We are willing to let you have some administrative flexibility, but we want a few guidelines. We want to have some results.

Dr. Edwards I think there might be some question as to whether these are guidelines or regulations.

Mr. Rogers We find the Congress very seldom writes regulations sufficient to really control the programs. We find those usually come from the Executive which sometimes pervert the law as stated. That is why these may seem a little more specific so that we can be sure it is very clear, the intent of the law, so that regulations will not change that intent. If you need discretion to include a little more, some of the low-impact areas, I think this committee would consider that. But this is the type of information we need:

Would you submit language for that?

Dr. Bataldan (*Director, Bureau of Community Health Services*) We certainly will.

Later in the hearings, some consumer representatives of in-stream projects, the East Coast Migrant Health Project, and the Migrant Legal Action Program (MLAP) testified in support of the bill, except for the concentration of funds provision. I myself was spontaneously called by Rogers from the audience to testify, and I restated the case for concentrating funds in as politic a manner as I could.

The clean bill, H.R. 14214 (see Appendix G), reported out of the subcommittee after markup on April 11, 1974, reflected the hearings. The mandate for comprehensiveness was watered down, or one could say administrative flexibility was added, by adding the words "as may be appropriate for particular centers" to the requirements for project services beyond primary care. High-impact areas were redefined by substituting a two-months residency for six months, the effect of which would be to increase the comprehensive sites by about one-third, by making eligible seven or eight counties in Michigan, and others in Washington, Oregon, Wisconsin, Ohio, etc. The percentage of funds to be devoted to the low-impact areas was raised to 20 percent. The funding level remained as before, but the provision for consumer input was weakened considerably by calling for "equitable representation of consumers of health services from the center, providers of health services, and the general public." This alteration was in response to the wishes of a conservative committee member; reportedly, Rogers made the alteration knowing that the HEW regulations were stronger and could be relied on.

A new provision was also added to the clean bill to the effect that a study be done on housing conditions of migrant workers, the effect of these conditions on health, and the role played by federal, state, and local standards. The Administration had reportedly suggested that a loan program for housing be authorized, but because that would cause conflict with the Department of Housing and Urban Development, Rogers substituted the fall-back position.

Although comprehensiveness, funds concentration, and consumer input were weakened, the funding level was retained and attractive provisions on environmental health and housing were added, and H.R. 14214 was still a recognizable relative of the original Shenkin-Biles draft.[d]

Meanwhile, Back in the Senate

Responsibility for the MHP in the Senate lay with Kennedy's aide for Chicano affairs, Mark Schneider, and with the professional staff of the Health Subcommittee. In the fall of 1972, they introduced a bill to extend the old legislation with four new provisions: (1) greatly increased funding up to $120 million in fiscal year 1975; (2) a special hospitalization fund with its own authorization up to $40 million in fiscal year 1975; (3) permission for the MHP to buy into ongoing HMOs on behalf of migrants; and (4) priority to be accorded consumer-based projects for awarding grants.

[d]On Monday, August 12, the next working day after President Nixon's resignation, the House passed H.R. 14214 by a vote of 359 to 12.

In the fall of 1973, they received technical aid from the MLAP and prepared a draft of a new bill in response to H.R. 11511. It altered 11511 basically by omitting the concept of concentrating funds on high-impact areas and recapitulating Kennedy's call for a special hospitalization fund and increased levels of general funding. Schneider asked for my comments in February, and I suggested concentrating funds, ensuring that projects reached a large size, targeting hospital funds to migrant center areas, and establishing three migrant advisory councils.

The Health Subcommittee worked over what Schneider gave them, and S. 3280 emerged on April 1. Its sixty-five pages dealt with community health centers, community mental health centers, and migrant health. The twenty-five pages of MHP consisted of an amalgam of the various proposals and some other programs, apparently. Comprehensiveness was mandated, concentration of funds was approached but not embraced, and consumer input was retained in projects but not mandated in the proposed structure of the National Advisory Council on Migrant Health Centers. Planning, development, construction, and hospitalization grants were authorized and given separate, generous funding; the general authorization was also high.

Other provisions seemed to thwart the bill's apparent basic intent. Great freedom was allowed in diluting a project's comprehensiveness and high priority was given existent projects. A provision requiring that projects not duplicate services in the local area would give project opponents a field day.

I was able to have more input into helping consumer and project administrator witnesses prepare their testimony for the May Senate hearings than I had had with the House. Also, the witnesses represented the home-base areas more equitably than before. Four major points were made by the witnesses before Kennedy, who was particularly attentive to the Chicano witnesses. They urged strengthening consumer input into project governing boards (compared with the House bill's provisions), concentrating money in high-impact areas, including a special hospitalization fund, and establishing three regional MHP advisory boards with predominant consumer representation.

After the hearings, Schneider requested that MLAP and I (we agreed with each other by now) draft language and supporting arguments for amending the House legislation in conference. Our major suggestions concerned the make-up of project governing boards, establishment of a MHP advisory committee, tightening the definition of high-impact areas, requiring projects to actively extend their services to all eligibles (in effect requiring large-sized projects), increasing regular funds, and establishing and funding a special hospital fund.

As of this writing (June 1974) the legislation still has not emerged from the subcommittee, and it appears inevitable that there will be a delay of months, past the expiration date of the legislation, before new legislation appears and is signed into law.

And at Appropriations . . .

It is instructive to read HEW's testimony before Chairman Flood of the House Labor-HEW Appropriations Subcommittee from March 21, 1974. Paul Bataldan, director of a newly enlarged Bureau of Community Health Services, testified that "We recognize that our main problem in terms of coverage for migrant health services is in the low-impact areas. We have migrant health services available in the high-impact areas of the country . . ." He pointed with pride to the number of visits the projects had recorded the previous year, and to subcommittee prodding, indicated that he had won a victory with OMB so the MHP funding could remain constant, and his major priority in the current year was to make the projects more efficient. This testimony was barely one month after HEW had testified to Rogers that they agreed with high-impact concentration of funds.

Appropriations is waiting for the authorizing legislation to be passed before they act.

CONCLUSION

The conclusions we can draw from the events of the past year and a half of legislative maneuvering are limited. I haven't done a great deal of independent investigation, but only recounted the events I was involved in, and the action is not yet concluded, although prospects do appear favorable. Some things can be said, however.

The duplicitous and insulting actions of the Nixon Administration in the health field, as well as Watergate, have produced a Congress much more amenable to specific legislation. I wanted specific legislation because of bureaucratic lethargy and priorities rather than political duplicity, but the coincidence in the world of politics has been beneficial.

Using the cloak of precedent proved a fruitful approach. Comprehensiveness was generally accepted as told in the words of the HMO bill; consumer participation was generally accepted and will emerge from conference, I think, as lifted from the regulations. Being able to use such tactics shows how incremental the basic approach was, and this too enhanced the chance of success.

I proved to be a fairly acceptable lobbyist. I think this can be accounted for by several factors; I had no obvious personal gains to make, so people felt I could be trusted. I was also trusted because of a prestigious educational background, experience with the program, and all the work I had put in on the obscure subject in question. The similarity of my age, background, and general life style with those of the aides with whom I dealt was also an important factor. But perhaps most importantly, there was an absence of competition. Both congressional aides and administration officials had more important things than the MHP to occupy their time, and the only other voluntary agent besides myself to give any prolonged attention to the MHP was the MLAP, with whom I eventually reached a common set of goals.

The story of this small effort to make some changes in a small program for less than one-half of one percent of the country's population is not yet finished. I guess some good will come of it all, but if it doesn't, there are no particular enemies of the migrants we can blame it on directly. There are indeed enemies (agribusiness et al.) that have put the migrants into a position where they are unfortunate enough to need a special health program, and keep them there by preventing union organization and lobbying in other areas. But for the malfunctioning of that special health program, and the problems of reforming it, I think we can only blame the competition of other health priorities.

Appendixes

Appendix A

Legislative History, Migrant Health Act

PUBLIC LAW 87-692
87th CONGRESS, S. 1130
SEPTEMBER 25, 1962

Be it enacted by the Senate and House of Representatives of the United States of America in Congress assembled, That title III of the Public Health Service Act (42 U.S.C., ch. 6A, subch. II) is amended by inserting at the end of part A thereof the following new section:

Grants for Family Health Service Clinics for Domestic Agricultural Migratory Workers

"Sec. 310. There are hereby authorized to be appropriated for the fiscal year ending June 30, 1963, the fiscal year ending June 30, 1964, and the fiscal year ending June 30, 1965, such sums not to exceed $3,000,000 for any year, as may be necessary, to enable the Surgeon General, (1) to make grants to public and other nonprofit agencies, institutions, and organizations for paying part of the cost of (i) establishing and operating family health service clinics for domestic agricultural migratory workers and their families, including training persons to provide services in the establishing and operating of such clinics, and (ii) special projects to improve health services for and the health conditions of domestic agricultural migratory workers and their families, including training persons to provide health services for or otherwise improve the health conditions of such migratory workers and their families, and (2) to encourage and cooperate in programs for the purpose of improving health services for or otherwise improving the health conditions of domestic agricultural migratory workers and their families."

PUBLIC LAW 89-109
89th CONGRESS, S. 510
AUGUST 5, 1965

Migratory Workers Health Services

Sec. 3. (a) Section 310 of the Public Health Service Act is amended by striking out "for the fiscal year ending June 1963, the fiscal year ending June 30, 1964, and the fiscal year ending June 30, 1965, such sums, not to exceed $3,000,000 for any year, as may be necessary" and inserting in lieu thereof "not to exceed $7,000,000 for the fiscal year ending June 30, 1966, $8,000,000 for the fiscal year ending June 30, 1967, and $9,000,000 for the fiscal year ending June 30, 1968."

(b) Such section is further amended by inserting "including necessary hospital care, and" immediately after "agricultural migratory workers and their families," in clause (1) (ii) of such section.

PUBLIC LAW 90-574
OCTOBER 15, 1968

Title II—Migratory Workers
Extension of Special Grants for Health of Migratory Workers

Sec. 201. Section 310 of the Public Health Service Act (42 U.S.C. 242h) is amended by striking out "and $9,000,000 for the fiscal year ending June 30, 1968" and inserting in lieu thereof "$9,000,000 each for the fiscal year ending June 30, 1968 and the next fiscal year, and $15,000,000 for the fiscal year ending June 30, 1970."

PUBLIC LAW 91-209
91st CONGRESS, H.R. 14733
MARCH 12, 1970

Be it enacted by the Senate and House of Representatives of the United States of America in Congress assembled, That section 310 of the Public Health Service Act (42 U.S.C. 242h) is amended—

(1) by striking out "and" after "next fiscal year,", and by inserting after "June 30, 1970," the following: "$20,000,000 for the fiscal year ending June 30, 1971, $25,000,000 for the fiscal year ending June 30, 1972, and $30,000,000 for the fiscal year ending June 30, 1973."

(2) by adding at the end thereof the following new sentence: "The Secretary may also use funds appropriated under this section to provide health services to persons (and their families) who perform seasonal agricultural services similar to the services performed by domestic agricultural migratory

workers if the Secretary finds that the provision of health services under this sentence will contribute to the improvement of the health conditions of such migratory workers and their families."

(3) by adding immediately after the sentence added by paragraph (2) the following new sentence: "For the purposes of assessing and meeting domestic migratory agricultural workers' health needs, developing necessary resources, and involving local citizens in the development and implementation of health care programs authorized by this section, the Secretary must be satisfied, upon the basis of evidence supplied by each applicant, that persons broadly representative of all elements of the population to be served and others in the community knowledgeable about such needs have been given an opportunity to participate in the development of such programs, and will be given an opportunity to participate in the implementation of such programs."

(4) by striking out "to improve health services for and the health conditions of" in clause (1) (ii) and inserting in lieu thereof "to improve and provide a continuity in health services for and to improve the health conditions of."

(5) by inserting "(including allied health professions personnel)" after "training persons" each place it appears in clause (1).

(6) (A) by striking out "Surgeon General" and inserting in lieu thereof "Secretary," and (B) by inserting at the beginning of such section the following heading: "Health Services for Domestic Agricultural Migrants."

Appendix B

Grants for Migrant Health Service—Rules and Regulations

TITLE 42—PUBLIC HEALTH

Chapter 1—Public Health Service, Department of Health, Education, and Welfare

Subchapter D—Grants

Part 56—Grants for Migrant Health Service

On December 28, 1971, proposed regulations concerning grants for migrant health services were published in the *Federal Register* (36 F.R. 25044, December 28, 1971) and public comment was invited. Approximately 200 comments were received. Although most comments were favorable, many were critical of particular provisions of the proposed regulations. In particular, concern was expressed that some State and local governmental agencies would not be able to establish Project Policy Boards under existing State law. In a similar vein, concern was expressed that existing grantees would not be able to change over from existing advisory-type boards to the required Project Policy Board within the time for filing applications for continuation grants. Although the requirement for the creation of the Project Policy Board will be retained, it has been determined that the regulations should be revised to permit a period for affected grantees to bring themselves into compliance.

In addition, the selection process with respect to membership on the Board has been amended to provide that 51 percent of the members of the Policy Board shall be chosen by the population to be served, eliminating the requirement that all such members must be from the population to be served.

Also, the requirement with respect to the creation of a separate Professional Advisory Committee has been deleted, because it was felt that separate boards and committees would not promote the desired cooperation and

From the *Federal Register* 37, 102 (May 25, 1972): 10646–49.

exchange between consumers and health professionals. Instead, the Project Policy Board will be required to have at least three members who are representatives of the community with knowledge of the health needs of the population to be served and experience in the delivery of health care services.

Many other comments discussed details of particular regulatory provisions or sought clarifications which will be dealt with in pending program guidelines.

Accordingly, having duly considered all comments received, the regulations as set forth below, are hereby adopted effective on the date of their publication in the *Federal Register* (5-25-72).

Dated: March 25, 1972.

Vernon E. Wilson,
Administrator, Health Services and Mental Health Administration.

Approved: April 17, 1972.
Elliot L. Richardson,
Secretary.

Sec.
56.101 Applicability.
56.102 Definitions.
56.103 Eligibility.
56.104 Application for grant.
56.105 Project Policy Board.
56.106 Project elements.
56.107 Grant evaluation and award.
56.108 Grant payments.
56.109 Use of project funds.
56.110 Civil rights.
56.111 Confidentiality.
56.112 Inventions or discoveries.
56.113 Publications and copyright.
56.114 Grantee accountability.
56.115 Records, reports, inspection, and audit.
56.116 Additional conditions.
56.117 Early termination and withholding of payments.

Authority: The provisions of this Part 56 issued under sec. 215, 58 Stat. 690, as amended; 42 U.S.C. 216; sec. 310, 76 Stat. 592, as amended; 42 U.S.C. 242h.

§56.101 Applicability. The regulations in this part are applicable to the award of grants under section 310 of the Public Health Service Act (42

U.S.C. 242h) for projects providing health services to, improving health services of, or otherwise improving the health conditions of, domestic agricultural migratory workers, seasonal agricultural workers, and their families.

§56.102 Definitions. As used in this part:

(a) "Act" means section 310 of the Public Health Service Act, as amended (42 U.S.C. 242h).

(b) "State" means any of the several States, the District of Columbia, Puerto Rico, and the Virgin Islands.

(c) "Secretary" means the Secretary of Health, Education, and Welfare and any other officer or employee of the Department of Health, Education, and Welfare to whom the authority involved has been delegated.

(d) "Domestic Agricultural Migratory Worker" means an individual residing in a State whose principal occupation is in agriculture on a seasonal basis, who establishes for the purpose of such employment a temporary place of abode and who has been so employed within the last 24 months.

(e) "Seasonal Agricultural Worker" means an individual residing in a State whose principal occupation is in agriculture on a seasonal basis, who has been so employed within the last 24 months and who has not established a temporary place of abode.

(f) "Agriculture" means farming in all its branches including but not limited to cultivation and tillage of the soil, the production, cultivation, growing, and harvesting of any commodity grown on, in or as an adjunct to or part of an item grown in or on the land including any practices performed by a farmer or on a farm as an incident to or in conjunction with such farming operations, including preparation for market, delivery to storage or to market or to carriers for transportation to market.

§56.103 Eligibility. (a) *Eligible applicants.* Any public or other nonprofit institution, agency, or organization is eligible for a grant award.

(b) *Eligible projects.* Grants may be made by the Secretary under the Act to pay part of the cost of a project:

(1) To establish and operate family health service clinics for domestic agricultural migratory workers and their families including training persons to provide services in the establishing and operating such clinics.

(2) To improve and provide a continuity in health services for, and to improve the health conditions of, domestic agricultural migratory workers and their families, including necessary hospital care, and including training persons to provide health services for or otherwise improve health conditions of such migratory workers and their families; or

(3) To provide health services to persons (and their families) who perform seasonal agricultural services similar to the services performed by domestic agricultural migratory workers if the Secretary finds that the project is

located in an area where migratory workers reside and the provision of such services will contribute to the improvement of the health conditions of such migratory workers and their families.

§56.104 Application for grant. (a) An application for a grant under this part shall be submitted to the Secretary in such form and manner and at such time as the Secretary may prescribe.

(b) The application shall contain a budget and a narrative plan of the manner in which the applicant intends to conduct the project and carry out the requirements of this part.

(c) Such application shall be executed by an individual authorized to act for the applicant and to assume on behalf of the applicant, the obligations imposed by the statute, and terms and conditions of any award, including the regulations of this part.

(d) Such application shall set forth the membership of the Project Policy Board (hereinafter referred to as the board) described in §56.105 and shall also be executed by the chairman or such other representative selected by the board, authorized to act for the board and to assume on its behalf the obligations imposed by the Act and by the terms and conditions of any award, and the regulations of this part. Such execution shall constitute the acceptance by the board of the terms and conditions of the grant and obligate it to perform its functions under the approved project in accordance with the terms thereof, the Act and the regulations of this part.

§56.105 Project Policy Board. (a) Except as provided in paragraph (b) of this section. Project Policy Board shall be established by an applicant as follows:

(1) *Size.* The board shall be sufficiently large to provide adequate participation by the population to be served and shall have its chairman or other such leadership elected by the members of the board.

(2) *Selection and composition.* At least 51 percent of the members of the board shall be chosen by a democratic process by the population to be served and at least three members shall be representatives of the community with knowledge of the health needs of the population to be served and experience in the delivery of health care services. All members of the board shall be selected to serve for a period of one year.

(3) *Meetings.* The board shall meet as often as necessary but not less than once a month during the time project services are being offered.

(4) *Functions.* (i) The board, after consultation with appropriate project staff shall from time to time establish, amend, and revise general policy in areas indicated in subdivision (ii) of this subparagraph with regard to the operation of the project: *Provided, however,* That in establishing such policy the board shall not—

(*a*) Establish any policy which is inconsistent with the Act or these regulations or which prevents the fulfillment of obligations imposed under the grant, or

(*b*) Involve itself in the day-to-day administration of the project, including the hiring or firing of any specific personnel except the project director, who shall be hired or fired only with the approval of the board.

(ii) The areas in which the board shall establish, amend, and revise general policy shall include at least the following:

(*a*) Selection and dismissal of personnel, including qualifications, salary and benefits, and grievance procedures;

(*b*) Selection and elimination of health care services;

(*c*) Eligibility for services;

(*d*) Hours and location of services;

(*e*) Priorities for allocation of project funds among services; and

(*f*) Methods of evaluating the project.

(b) The Secretary may, for good cause shown, allow a grantee a period of time for compliance with the requirements of these regulations with respect to the board as follows:

(1) *Continuation grants.* A grantee under a continuation grant may be given a reasonable period of time, not to exceed 1 year from the effective date of these regulations, to establish a board meeting the requirements of paragraph (a) of this section.

(2) *Inconsistent State or local law.* In addition, in the case of a grantee which is a State or local governmental agency and which has demonstrated to the satisfaction of the Secretary that it is unable, under State or local law, to establish a board pursuant to paragraph (a) of this section, the Secretary may allow such grantee a reasonable period of time to take the appropriate steps to have such legal disability removed. *Provided* That, such grantee, in the interim, must establish alternate procedures, approved by the Secretary, to assure maximum participation in the development, implementation, and evaluation of the project by the population to be served consistent with the concept of a Project Policy Board as set forth in paragraph (a) of this section. Nothing in this paragraph shall relieve an applicant of the requirements of §56.106(a) (2).

§56.106 Project elements. (a) An approvable application must provide:

(1) That all project elements will be provided in a manner calculated to preserve human dignity and to maximize acceptability and utilization of services.

(2) That persons broadly representative of all elements of the population to be served and others in the community knowledgeable about such needs have been given an opportunity to participate in the development of

such program and will be given an opportunity to participate in the implementation and evaluation of such program.

(3) That the project will deliver or arrange for the delivery of family-oriented primary health care which shall include, but not be limited to:

(i) Ambulatory patient diagnosis, treatment, and followup care for acute and chronic conditions:

(ii) Preventive, maternal, child health, and family planning services integrated into the delivery of treatment services:

(iii) Emergency medical and dental care; and

(iv) Diagnostic, preventive, and basic restorative dental care.

(4) That the project has established a system for maintaining health services records.

(5) That the project will arrange for:

(i) Referral of complex, difficult, or unusual cases and adequate followup to insure continuity of care;

(ii) Hospitalization of patients and hospital staff privileges for project physicians; and

(iii) Transportation, if required for patient care.

(6) That no person shall be denied service by reason of his inability to pay therefor: *Provided, however,* That a charge for the provision of services will be made to the extent that a third party (including a Government agency) is authorized or is under legal obligation to pay such charge: *And further provided,* That where the cost of care and services furnished by or through the project is to be reimbursed under title XIX of the Social Security Act, a written agreement with the title XIX agency is required.

(7) That subject to the provisions of subparagraph (6) of this paragraph, charges to be made for services rendered pursuant to the project, must be in accordance with a schedule submitted and approved as part of the project. Such schedule may provide for services to be rendered on a prepaid capitation basis. In those cases in which the project will provide services by contract or other similar arrangement with the actual providers of services, a plan shall be provided establishing rates and methods of payment (including payment on a prepaid capitation basis) for medical care. Such payment must be made pursuant to agreements with a schedule of rates, and payment procedures maintained by the grantee. The grantee must be prepared to substantiate that such rates are reasonable and necessary.

(8) That a Project Policy Board will be established in accordance with §56.105; and

(9) That the project shall provide and implement methods of evaluating the performance of activities being carried out under the grant to assure that such activities are carried out in accordance with the regulations of this part.

(b) An approvable application must also include the following elements unless the Secretary determines that the applicant has established good cause for their omission:

(1) That in developing and operating the project, arrangements have been made for the provision of the following ancillary services: Nutrition, respiratory disease care, accident prevention, environmental health services, and health and sanitation education;

(2) That paramedical and allied health professional personnel have been or will be employed by the project; and

(3) That a plan for education of the population to be served as to the availability and location of supplementary health facilities and services has been or will be developed.

§56.107 Grant evaluation and award. (a) Within the limits of funds available for such purpose, the Secretary may award grants to cover part of the cost of projects to those applicants whose projects will in his judgment best promote the purposes of the Act taking into account.

(1) The overall significance of the project in terms of the numbers of persons served, the relative need to be met, the duration of services to be provided, and the general quality of the project's plan in accordance with the project elements cited in §56.106;

(2) The administrative and management capability and competence of the applicant:

(3) The competence of the staff in relation to the services to be provided;

(4) The extent to which the project will provide a continuity of patient care; and

(5) The comments and evaluations of the population to be served relative to the proposed project.

(b) The amount of any award shall be determined by the Secretary on the basis of his estimate of the sum necessary for all or a designated portion of direct project costs plus an additional amount for indirect costs, if any, which will be calculated by the Secretary either (1) on the basis of his estimate of the actual indirect costs reasonably related to the project, or (2) on the basis of a percentage of all, or a portion of, the estimated direct costs of the project when there are reasonable assurances that the use of such percentage will not exceed the approximate actual indirect costs. Such award may include an estimated provisional amount for indirect costs or for designated direct costs (such as hospital per diem rates or fringe benefit rates) subject to upward (within the limits of available funds) as well as downward adjustments to actual costs when the amount properly expended by the grantee for provisional items has been determined by the Secretary: *Provided, however,* That no grant shall be made for an amount equal to the total cost as found necessary by the Secretary for the carrying out of the project. In determining the grantee's share of project costs, costs for which Federal grants from other sources have been or may be claimed or received or costs used to match other Federal grants except as may be otherwise provided by law, or costs to be met from the Federal share of grant related income (except as may be permitted by chapter 1-420 of the Department of Health, Education, and Welfare Grants Administration Manual[1]) may not be included.

(c) Except as may otherwise be provided by the regulations of this part, the identification of direct and indirect costs will be consistent with the generally accepted and established accounting practices that the grantee applies to its own activities and in conformance with the applicable principles set forth in chapters 1-76, 2-65, 2-66, and 5-60 of the Department of Health, Education, and Welfare Grants Administration Manual.

(d) All grant awards shall be in writing, shall set forth the amount of funds granted and the period for which support is recommended.

(e) Neither the approval of any project nor any grant award shall commit or obligate the United States in any way to make any additional, supplemental, continuation, or other award with respect to any approved project or portion thereof. For continuation support, grantees must make separate applications annually at such times and in such form as the Secretary may direct.

§ 56.108 Grant payments. The Secretary shall from time to time make payments to a grantee of all or a portion of any grant award, either in advance or by way of reimbursement for expenses incurred or to be incurred in the performance of the project to the extent he determines such payments necessary to promote prompt initiation and advancement of the approved project. Such payments may include reimbursement to a grantee for services rendered on a prepaid capitation basis.

§56.109 Use of project funds. (a) Any funds granted pursuant to this part as well as other funds to be used in performance of the approved project shall be expended solely for carrying out the approved project in accordance with the statute, the regulations of this part, the terms and conditions of the award and cost principles set forth in the Department of Health, Education, and Welfare Grants Administration Manual.

(b) Project funds may be used to reimburse members of the Project Policy Board for actual expenses: *Provided,* That Domestic Agricultural Migra-

1. The Department Grants Administration Manual is available for inspection at the Public Information Office of the several Department Regional Offices and available for purchase at the Government Printing Office, GPO Document No. 894-523.

tory Workers and Seasonal Agricultural Workers may also be reimbursed for wages lost by reason of attendance at meetings.

(c) Prior approval by the Secretary of revision of the budget and project plan is required whenever there is to be a significant change in the scope or nature of project activities.

§ 56.110 Civil rights. Attention is called to the requirements of title VI of the Civil Rights Act of 1964 (78 Stat. 252, 42 U.S.C. 2000d et seq.) and in particular section 601 of such Act which provides that no person in the United States shall on the grounds of race, color, or national origin be excluded from participation in, be denied the benefits of, or be subjected to discrimination under any program or activity receiving Federal financial assistance. A regulation implementing such title VI, which applies to grants made under this part, has been issued by the Secretary of Health, Education, and Welfare with the approval of the President (45 CFR Part 80). In addition, no person shall on the grounds of age, sex, creed, or marital status (unless otherwise medically indicated) be excluded from participation in, be denied the benefits of, or be subjected to discrimination under any program or activity receiving Federal financial assistance. Nor shall any person be denied employment in or by such program or activity so receiving Federal financial assistance on the grounds of age, sex, creed, or marital status.

§56.111 Confidentiality. Each grant award is subject to the condition that all information obtained by the personnel of the project from participants in the project related to their examination, care, and treatment, shall be held confidential, and shall not be divulged without the individual's consent except as may be required by law or as may be necessary to provide service to the individual. Information may be disclosed in summary, statistical, or other form which does not identify particular individuals.

§56.112 Inventions or discoveries. Any grant award pursuant to §56.107 is subject to the regulations of the Department of Health, Education, and Welfare as set forth in 45 CFR Parts 6 and 8, as amended. Such regulations shall apply to any activity for which grant funds are in fact used whether within the scope of the project as approved or otherwise. Appropriate measures shall be taken by the grantee and by the Secretary to assure that no contracts, assignments or other arrangements inconsistent with the grant obligation are continued or entered into and that all personnel involved in the supported activity are aware of and comply with such obligations. Laboratory notes, related technical data, and information pertaining to inventions and discoveries shall be maintained for such periods, and filed with or otherwise made available to the Secretary, or those he may designate at such times and in such manner, as he may determine necessary to carry out such Department regulations.

§56.113 Publications and copyright. Except as may otherwise be provided under the terms and conditions of the award, the grantee may copyright without prior approval any publications, films or similar materials developed or resulting from a project supported by a grant under this part, subject, however, to a royalty-free, nonexclusive, and irrevocable license or right in the Government to reproduce, translate, publish, use, disseminate, and dispose of such materials and to authorize others to do so.

§56.114 Grantee accountability. (a) *Accounting for grant award payments.* All payments made by the Secretary shall be recorded by the grantee in accounting records separate from the records of all other grant funds, including funds derived from other grant awards. With respect to each approved project the grantee shall account for the sum total of all amounts paid by presenting or otherwise making available evidence satisfactory to the Secretary of expenditures for direct and indirect costs meeting the requirements of this part: *Provided, however,* That when the amount awarded for indirect cost was based on a predetermined fixed-percentage of estimated direct costs, the amount allowed for indirect costs shall be computed on the basis of such predetermined fixed-percentage rates applied to the total, or a selected element thereof, of the reimbursable direct costs incurred.

(b) *Accounting for equipment.* As used in this section the term "equipment" means an article of property procured or fabricated which is complete in itself, is of a durable nature, and has an expected service life of more than 1 year. Equipment on hand on the date of termination for which accounting is required in accordance with the procedures set forth in chapter 1-410-50 of the Department of Health, Education, and Welfare Grants Administration Manual shall be identified and reported by the grantee in accordance with such procedures, and, accounted for by one or a combination of the following methods, as determined by the Secretary:

(1) *Retention of equipment for other migrant health projects.* Equipment may be used, without adjustment of accounts, on other grant supported projects (whether or not federally supported) within the scope of the Act, and no other accounting for such equipment shall be required: *Provided, however,* (i) That during such period of use no charge for depreciation, amortization, or for other use of the equipment shall be made against any existing or future Federal grant or contract, and (ii) if, within the period of its useful life, the equipment is transferred by sale or otherwise for use outside the scope of the Act, the Federal portion of the fair market value at the time of transfer shall be refunded to the Federal Government.

(2) *Sale or other disposition of equipment, crediting of proceeds or value.* The equipment may be sold by the grantee and the net proceeds of the sale credited to the grant account for project use, or they may be used or disposed of in any manner by the grantee by crediting to the grant account the

Federal share of the fair market value on the termination date. To the extent equipment purchased from grant funds is used for credit or trade-in on the purchase of new equipment, the accounting obligation shall apply to the same extent to such new equipment.

(3) *Return or transfer of equipment.* The equipment may be returned to the Federal Government by the grantee or, in accordance with the provisions of chapter 1-410-50B of the Department of Health, Education, and Welfare Grants Administration Manual may be transferred to another grantee for the purpose of continuing the project for which the equipment was purchased.

(c) *Accounting for grant related income*—(1) *Interest.* Pursuant to section 203 of the Intergovernmental Cooperation Act of 1968 (42 U.S.C. 4213), a State will not be held accountable for interest earned on grant funds, pending their disbursement for grant purposes. A State, as defined in section 102 of the Intergovernmental Cooperation Act, means any one of the several States, the District of Columbia, Puerto Rico, any territory or possession of the United States, or any agency or instrumentality of a State, but does not include the governments of the political subdivisions of the State. All grantees other than a State, as defined in this subsection, must return all interest earned on grant funds to the Federal Government.

(2) *Royalties.* Royalties earned from publications or similar material produced from a grant must first be used to reduce the Federal share of the grant to cover the costs of publishing or producing the materials. Royalties in excess of the costs of publishing or producing the materials shall be distributed as in subparagraph (3) of this paragraph.

(3) *Other income.* Other income earned by the grantee shall be disposed of in accordance with one of the alternatives specified in chapter 1-420 of the Grants Administration Manual as determined by the Secretary in the grant award.

(d) *Grant closeout*—(1) *Date of final accounting.* A grantee shall render, with respect to each approved project, a full account, as provided herein, as of date of the termination of grant support. The Secretary may require other special and periodic accounting.

(2) *Final settlement.* There shall be payable to the Federal Government as final settlement with respect to each approved project the total sum of:

(i) Any amount not accounted for pursuant to paragraph (a) of this section;

(ii) Any credits for material on hand as provided in paragraph (b) of this section;

(iii) Any credits for earned interest pursuant to paragraph (c) (1) of this section;

(iv) Any other settlements required pursuant to paragraph (c) (2) and (3) of this section.

Such total sum shall constitute a debt owed by the grantee to the Federal Government and shall be recovered from the grantee or its successors or assignees by set off or other action as provided by law.

§56.115 Records, reports, inspection, and audit. (a) *Records and reports.* Each grant awarded pursuant to this part shall be subject to the condition that the grantee shall maintain such operational and accounting records, identifiable by grant number, and file with the Secretary such operational and fiscal reports relating to the use of grant funds, as the Secretary may find necessary to carry out the purposes of the Act and the regulations. All records shall be retained for 3 years after the close of the budget period. Such records may be destroyed at the end of such 3-year period if the applicant has been notified of the completion of the Federal audit by such time. If the applicant has not been so notified, such records shall be retained (1) for 5 years after the close of the budget period or (2) until the grantee is notified of the completion of the Federal audit, whichever comes first. In all cases where audit questions have arisen before the expiration of such 5-year period, records shall be retained until resolution of all such question.

(b) *Inspection and audit.* Any application for a grant under this part shall constitute the consent of the applicant to inspections of the facilities, equipment, and other resources of the applicant at reasonable times by persons designated by the Secretary and to interview with principal staff members to the extent that such resources and personnel are, or will be, part of the project. In addition, the acceptance of any grant under this part shall constitute the consent of the grantee to inspections and fiscal audits by such persons of the supported activity and of records relating to the use of grant funds.

§56.116 Additional conditions. The Secretary may with respect to any grant award impose additional conditions prior to or at the time of any award when in his judgment such conditions are necessary to assure or protect advancement of the approved project, the interests of public health, or the conservation of grant funds.

§56.117 Early termination and withholding of payments. Whenever the Secretary finds that a grantee has failed in a material respect to comply with the Act, the regulations of this part, or the terms of the grant, he may, on reasonable notice to the grantee, withhold further payments, and take such other action, including the termination of the grant, as he finds appropriate to carry out the purposes of the Act and regulations. Noncancelable obligations of the grantee properly incurred prior to the receipt of the notice of termination will be honored. The grantee shall be promptly notified of such termination in writing and given the reasons therefor.

[FR Doc. 72-7975 Filed 5-24-72; 8:55 am]

Appendix C

Migrant Impact Settings

Migrant Impact Settings by Location, Type, and Number of Migrants (4,000 or more migrants and dependents)

State	*County*	*Total Migrants and Dependents*
I. *Home-Base Settings*–Counties with resident migrants and few non-resident in-migrants.		
California	Imperial	10,420
Florida	Orange	7,250
	Polk	6,300
	Seminole	12,850
New Mexico	Rio Arriba	4,200
	San Miguel	10,000
Texas	Bexar	11,000
	Cameron	28,540
	Castro	4,700
	Deaf Smith	10,000
	Hale	7,200
	Hidalgo	45,000
	Lamb	4,020
	Lubbock	7,792
	Maverick	9,600
	Nueces	5,000
	San Patricio	4,392
	Starr	4,285
	Val Verde	4,425
	Webb	9,993
	Zavala*	7,000
II. *Mixed Settings*–Counties with many resident farm workers and substantial employment of in-migrants.		
Arizona	Maricopa	16,671
	Pinal	20,000

State	*County*	*Total Migrants and Dependents*
California	Fresno	56,000
	Kern	22,100
	Merced	7,200
	Monterey	8,970
	Riverside	7,100
	San Joaquin	13,790
	Sutter	4,000
	Stanislaus	9,740
	Tulare	23,110
	Ventura	7,250
	Yolo	4,530
Florida	Broward	14,000
	Collier	18,900
	Dade	17,500
	Glades-Hendry	10,500
	Lee	9,000
	Palm Beach	38,358
Washington	Skagit	10,350
	Yakima	20,404

III. *Upstream Settings*—Counties with substantial in-migration of workers, but with small resident migrant population.

State	*County*	*Total Migrants and Dependents*	
		Brief Duration	*Medium Duration*
Arkansas	White	4,200	
Colorado	Weld		7,000
Connecticut	Hartford		6,100
Michigan	Allegan		7,772
	Berrien		27,790
	Grand Traverse		9,506
	Oceana		4,640
	Van Buren		37,302
New Jersey	Cumberland		4,139
New Mexico	Dona Ana		4,000
Ohio	Sandusky		11,000
Oregon	Marion		10,700
South Carolina	Charleston	4,395	
Washington	Douglas-Chelan	4,910	
	Okanogan	6,084	
Wisconsin	Door		4,900
	Waushara		8,700

Source: Community Change, Inc., modifying 1969 Senate Subcommittee on Migratory Labor estimates by using 1970 and 1971 data from State health and employment agencies in California, Florida, Michigan, Texas and Washington.

Appendix D

Sampling of Projects from the Classical Migrant Health Program

In 1971 the author abstracted information from twenty-five "classical" projects selected for size; Eastern, Western, or Central stream; home base or upstream location; sponsorship; and state. Both annual reports and budgets were reviewed, mostly from the year 1969, but some from 1968 when the 1969 file was not available. The information derived is related in the figures and tables referring to Chapter 3. The sample projects reflected all MHP projects then current (excluding the state-level consulting grants) as follows:

	Sample projects		*All projects*
Number of projects	25		137
Number of states represented	14		37
Location:			
home base	10	(40%)	(31%)
up-stream	15	(60%)	(69%)
Sponsorship:			
home base—health dept.	7	(70%)	(77%)
local gov't.	2	(20%)	(9%)
medical society	1	(10%)	(5%)
upstream—health dept.	6	(40%)	(63%)
vol. agency	5	(33%)	(21%)
local gov't.	7	(20%)	(10%)
medical society	1	(7%)	(3%)
Size:			
home base—less than $60,000 annual budget	7	(70%)	(57%)
greater than $60,000 annual budget	3	(30%)	(43%)

upstream–less than $60,000 annual budget	13	(87%)	(75%)
greater than $60,000 annual budget	2	(13%)	(25%)

Appendix E

Migrant Health Program, Current Operations and Additional Needs

Health Services Assisted by Migrant Health Grants
Distribution of Grant Dollars by Type of Service 1963–1967

		Distribution	
Fiscal Year	*Grant Funds Available and Awarded*	*Personal Health Care Percent*	*Sanitation Services Percent*
1963	$ 750,000	91	9
1964	1,500,000	91	9
1965	2,500,000	90	10
1966	3,000,000	90	10
1967	7,200,000	90	10
	$14,950,000	90	10

From "Migrant Health Program, Current Operations and Additional Needs," pp. 22, 25, 26, and 28.

This report was made by the Public Health Service and transmitted to the Committee on Labor and Public Welfare of the Senate. It was then printed for the use of the Committee by Government Printing Office, Washington, 1967.

Health Services Offered by Grant-Assisted Migrant Health Projects During 1966; Estimated Projections for 1967 and 1968

	1966	*1967 estimate*	*1968 estimate*
Migrants:			
Total number, United States	1,000,000	1,000,000	1,000,000
Number in project areas at some time during year	250,000	300,000	350,000
Counties with migrant influx:			
Total number, United States	726	726	726
Number offering grant-assisted services:			
Personal health and sanitation (combined)	270	280	300
Sanitation only	142	150	150
Personal health services provided migrants:[1]			
Medical visits	165,000	215,000	265,000
Dental visits	18,000	24,000	30,000
Hospital patients	0	4,200	5,700
Hospital patient days	0	29,400	39,900
Nursing visits to camps, etc.	100,000	125,000	150,000
Sanitary inspections and followup visits	100,000	125,000	150,000
Appropriation:			
Health service support	$3,000,000	$7,200,000	$8,100,000
Consultation and program tools	$500,000	$800,000	$800,000

1. Health education is potentially a part of every service. Data are not separately reported.

HEALTH SERVICE DEFICIENCIES – JANUARY 1967

MIGRANT-IMPACT COUNTIES LACKING GRANT-ASSISTED HEALTH SERVICES

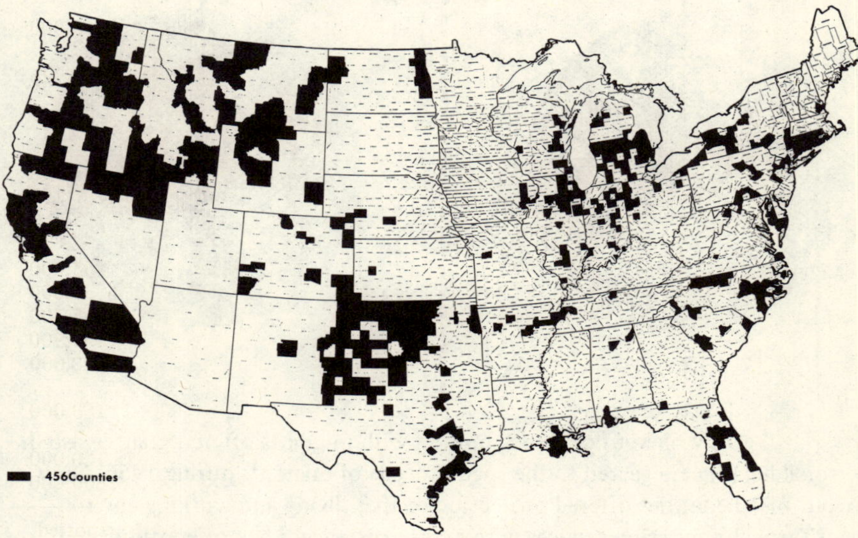

For continuity of health care and protection, migrants need access to health services in every county where they live and work temporarily. Because geographic coverage by project services is still far from complete, a total of 750,000 migrants had no access to personal health care provided through projects in 1966. The remainder had ready access to personal health services for only part of the year.

HEALTH SERVICE DEFICIENCIES

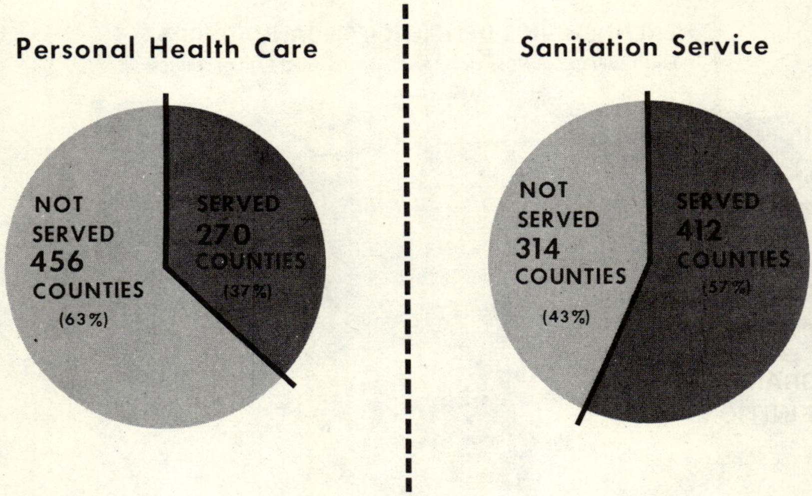

Only one out of three counties with migrants offered grant-assisted personal health care geared to the special needs of migrants during 1966. Only six out of 10 counties offered protection of their living and working environment through sanitation services with grant assistance. Lack of continuity of health care will remain a problem as long as many communities have no place to which a migrant can turn and expect to find needed health care.

Appendix F

Shenkin-Biles Draft of Proposed Legislation, February 1973

MIGRANT HEALTH CENTERS DEFINITIONS

"Sec. 1. Definitions for the purposes of this title:

"(1) The term 'migrant health organization' means a public or non-profit private entity which—

"(A) provides primary health services directly in one or more migrant health centers and arranges supplemental health services for all of the residents of a migrant impacted area;

"(B) provides for all of the residents of the area (i) environmental health services including the detection and alleviation of unhealthful conditions of water supply, sewage treatment, solid waste disposal, pest infestation, field sanitation, and other environmental factors related to health; (ii) infectious and parasitic disease screening and control; and (iii) accident prevention including prevention of excessive pesticide exposure;

"(C) actively provides for residents of the area information on the availability of and proper utilization of health services;

"(D) has organizational arrangements for an ongoing quality assurance program which stresses both health service processes and outcomes and assures that health services provided meet standards established in accordance with regulations of the Secretary;

"(E) assures that the primary and supplemental health services are available and accessible to all the residents of the area promptly and appropriately and in a manner which assures continuity; services, as appropriate, shall be available to residents on a 24-hour basis;

"(F) demonstrates its financial responsibility by the use of accepted accounting procedures and otherwise maintaining a generally solvent operation;

"(G) provides an effective procedure for developing, compiling, evaluating and reporting to the Secretary data (which the Secretary shall publish and disseminate on a periodic basis) relating to (i) the health status of persons residing in the area; (ii) the patterns of utilization of center services; (iii) the availability, accessibility and acceptability of center services; (iv) the effect of center services on the health of residents; and (v) the costs of center operations presented on both a line item and programmatic basis;

"(H) is directed by a board of directors that (i) has at least a majority of its members directly selected in a democratic manner by the enrolled members of the center; when the center is in the planning and development period, representatives of organized consumer groups whose members are primarily migrants from the area may substitute for the directly selected members; (ii) meets at least once a month; (iii) explicitly directs general policy in the following areas (a) employment of the project director; (b) establishment of personnel policies; (c) selection of health services to be offered; (d) establishment of payment schedules; (e) establishment of locations and hours of service; (iv) approves the annual budget and significant changes in the budget; (v) keeps minutes which are openly available to the media and the public.

"(2) The term 'primary health services' means the following services provides in an ambulatory setting:

"(A) physician services;

"(B) diagnostic laboratory and radiologic services;

"(C) preventive, maternal, child health, and family planning services;

"(D) emergency medical services;

"(E) emergency dental care and basic preventive dental care for residents under five (5) years of age; and

"(F) transportation services as required for adequate patient care.

"(3) The term 'supplemental health services' means

"(A) in-patient hospital services;

"(B) home health services;

"(C) rehabilitation services; and

"(D) physician services for complex, difficult or unusual cases.

"(4) The term 'migrant' means an individual residing in a State whose principal occupation is in agriculture on a seasonal basis, who establishes for the purpose of such employment a temporary place of abode and who has been so employed within the last 24 months.

"(5) The term 'migrant health center' means an institution for the provision of health care which:

"(A) is primarily located at a single geographical site (a center may operate subsidiary satellite centers as necessary to provide services to the residents of the area);

"(B) has at least five full time physicians;

"(C) has a unitary and integrated budget;

"(D) functions under a single administration; and

"(E) maintains unified medical and other record systems.

"(6) The term 'migrant impacted area' means a geographic area, contiguous, (except for the inclusion of proximal migrant pockets of population), of reasonable size for health delivery from a central source, in which reside for at least five months per year at least eight thousand migrants and in which reside from 10,000 to 25,000 persons in all.

"Sec. 2. Planning and Development.

"(1) The Secretary may make grants subject to the general provisions of this title to public or private non-profit entities to assist in projects for the planning and development of migrant health organizations. No project may receive more than $250,000 in grants under this section. Funds awarded under such grants shall be available for expenditure by the grantee for a period not to exceed one year from the date of award.

"(2) The Secretary in making grants under this section shall give priority to those entities which demonstrate that assistance and consultation in the planning and developing will be provided by individuals and organizations with previous experience and expertise in the comprehensive health systems field.

"(3) Sums awarded under such grant shall be utilized for purposes including, but not limited to:

"(A) implementation of a consumer acquaintance campaign including election of representatives;

"(B) detail, design of, and arrangements for the health services to be provided;

"(C) development of the administrative and internal organizational arrangements including fiscal control and fund accounting procedures;

"(D) recruitment of personnel and the conduct of personnel training activities; and

"(E) payment of architects' and engineers' fee."

"Sec. 3. Operational Grants

"(1) The Secretary may make grants, subject to the provisions of this title, to migrant health organizations to assist them in meeting their costs of operation; no organization may receive more than $2 1/2 million in grants in any year under this section.

"(2) In order to receive funds under this section, a migrant health center must provide reasonable assurance to the Secretary that the migrant health organization

"(A) has a contractual or other arrangement with the agency, of each state in which it provides services, which administers or supervises the administration of a state plan approved under title XIX of the Social Security Act under which arrangement all or a part of the basic health services payment required by the migrant health center is paid for its members who are eligible for medical assistance under such a state plan, or has made every reasonable effort to enter into such an arrangement; and

"(B) has made and will continue to make every reasonable effort to collect appropriate reimbursement for its costs in providing basic and supplemental health services to its members who are entitled to insurance benefits under title XVIII of such Act, to medical assistance under a state plan approved under title XIX of such Act, or to assistance for medical expenses under any other public assistance program or prive health insurance program."

"Sec. 4. Construction Grants

"(1) The Secretary may make grants, subject to the general provisions of this title, to any migrant health organization, or any entity intending to become a migrant health organization, to assist it in meeting the cost of construction of facilities for ambulatory services for the provisions of health services; the Secretary shall give special consideration to applications for grants for the acquisition or renovation of existing facilities; no grant under this section for any project may exceed 90 per centum of the cost of construction (as determined by the Secretary) of such project; no project may receive more than $2,500,000 in grants under this section."

"Sec. 5. Other Grants

"(1) There shall be established an 'upstream services fund', which may be used for the following purposes:

"(A) funding of coordination projects for the purposes of (i) helping migrants receive emergency care in areas where they are predominantly non-residents, and (ii) helping migrants with chronic illnesses under treatment at migrant health centers to receive proper follow-up care while in an area which does not have a migrant health center.

"(B) reimbursement for emergency medical and chronic illness followup services rendered to migrants in areas not served by migrant health centers."

"Sec. 6. Advisory Councils

"(1) There shall be established an eastern migrant council, a midcontinent migrant council, and a western migrant council to deal with the eastern, midcontinent and western migrant streams, respectively; each council shall be composed of six members appointed by the Secretary (without regard to the provisions of title 5 of the United States Code relating to appointments in the competitive service) from persons who are not officers or employees of the United States Government, and who including representatives of organized migrant groups, employers of migrants, migrant health organizations, and providers of health care to migrants; at least two members shall be migrants, and one at least shall be a physician; the Secretary shall appoint a chairman for each council.

"(2) Each member of the council shall hold office for a term of three years, except that

"(A) any member appointed to fill a vacancy prior to the expiration of the term for which his predecessor was appointed shall hold office for the remainder of such term, and

"(B) the terms of office of the members first taking office shall expire, as designated by the Secretary at the time of appointment, as follows: Three shall expire at the end of the first year, three at the end of the second year, and three at the end of the third year, after the date of appointment; a member shall not be eligible to service continuously for more than two terms.

"(3) Members of the council, while attending meetings or conferences thereof, or otherwise serving on business of the council, shall be entitled to receive compensation at rates fixed by the Secretary, but not exceeding for any days the daily equivalent of the effective rate for grade GS-18 of the general schedule, including travel time, and while so serving away from their homes or regular places of business, they may be allowed travel expenses, including per diem in lieu of subsistence, as authorized by section 5703(b) of title 5 of the United States Code for persons in government service employed intermittently.

"(4) The councils shall advise and assist the Secretary in the development of policy and preparation of regulations relating to programs under this title; the council shall consider applications for grants, loans, loan guarantees, and interest subsidy payments under this title and shall make recommendations to the Secretary with respect to approval of applications for assistance under this title and to amounts of grants, loans, and loan guarantees under this title."

"Sec. 7. Authorization of Funds

"(1) There are authorized to be appropriated for the purposes of this act $30,000,000 in fiscal year 1974; $50,000,000 in 1975, and $55,000,000 in 1976.

"(2) Of the funds appropriated under this Title no more than 15% shall be used to support the upstream services fund."

Appendix G

H.R. 14214, April 11, 1974

TITLE IV–MIGRANT HEALTH

Sec. 401. Section 310 of the Public Health Service Act is amended to read as follows:

"Health Services for Agricultural Migrants

"Sec. 310. (a) (1) For purposes of this section, the term 'migrant health center' means an entity which–

"(A) provides, in the manner prescribed by paragraph (2), the services described in such paragraph to–

"(i) agricultural migratory workers and their families, and

"(ii) persons in the area served by the entity who perform seasonal agricultural services similar to the services performed by agricultural migratory workers and their families if the Secretary finds that the provision of such services to such persons may contribute to the improvement of the health conditions of agricultural migratory workers and their families, and

"(B) is organized in the manner prescribed by paragraph (3).

"(2) A migrant health center shall provide each of the following:

"(A) Primary health services,

"(B) As may be appropriate for particular centers, supplemental health services necessary for the adequate support of primary health services,

"(C) Referral to providers of supplemental health services and payment, as appropriate and feasible, for their provision of such services,

"(D) Environmental health services, including, as may be appropriate for particular centers, the detection and alleviation of unhealthful conditions associated with water supply, sewage treatment, solid waste disposal, rodent and parasitic infestation, field sanitation, housing, and other environmental factors related to health,

"(E) As may be appropriate for particular centers, infectious and parasitic disease screening and control,

"(F) As may be appropriate for particular centers, accident prevention, including prevention of excessive pesticide exposure, and

"(G) Information on the availability and proper use of health services.

The services of a center shall be provided directly through its staff and supporting resources or through contracts or cooperative arrangements with public or private entities. Primary health services shall be available and accessible in the area served by the center promptly, as appropriate, and in a manner which assures continuity.

"(3) (A) The governing body of a migrant health center shall meet at least once a month, shall establish general policies for the center, shall approve the center's annual budget, and shall approve the selection of a director for the center. The composition and the manner of selection of the members of the governing body of a migrant health center shall be prescribed by regulations of the Secretary, except that there shall be on the governing body of a center an equitable representation of consumers of health services from the center, providers of health services, and the general public.

"(B) The center shall have organizational arrangements, established in accordance with regulations prescribed by the Secretary, for (i) an ongoing quality assurance program (including utilization and peer review systems) respecting the center's services, and (ii) maintaining the confidentiality of patient records.

"(b) For purposes of this section:

"(1) The term 'agricultural migratory worker' means an individual whose principal employment is employment in agriculture on a seasonal basis, who has been so employed within the last twenty-four months, and who establishes for the purpose of such employment a temporary abode.

"(2) The term 'primary health services' means—

"(A) services of physicians and, where feasible, services of physicians' assistants and nurse clinicians;

"(B) diagnostic laboratory and radiologic services;

"(C) preventive health services (including children's eye examinations to determine the need for vision correction, peri-natal services, well child services, and family planning services);

"(D) emergency medical services;

"(E) transportation services as required for adequate patient care; and

"(F) preventive dental services.

"(3) The term 'supplemental health services' means services which are not included as primary health services and which are—

"(A) hospital services;

"(B) home health services;
"(C) extended care facility services;
"(D) rehabilitation services;
"(E) dental services;
"(F) mental health services;
"(G) vision services;
"(H) allied health services;
"(I) pharmaceutical services;
"(J) health education services; and
"(K) services which promote and facilitate optimal use of primary health services and the services referred to in the preceding subparagraphs of this paragraph.

"(4) The term 'high impact area' means a county or other political subdivision within a State which has not less than six thousand agricultural migratory workers residing within its boundaries for more than two months in any calendar year.

"(c) The Secretary may make grants to public and nonprofit private entities to assist in (1) the establishment and initial operation of migrant health centers which will serve one or more high impact areas, and (2) meeting the costs of the continued operation of migrant health centers serving one or more such areas, including training related to the provision of primary, supplemental, and environmental health services and program management.

"(d) The Secretary may make grants to public and nonprofit private entities, and may enter into contracts with public and private entities, in areas in which no migrant health centers exist and which are not high impact areas—

"(1) for the provision of emergency care to agricultural workers and their families;

"(2) for the provision of primary care (as defined in regulations of the Secretary) for agricultural workers and their families;

"(3) for the development of arrangements with existing facilities to provide primary health services (not included as primary care as defined under regulations under paragraph (2)) to agricultural workers and their families, or

"(4) for activities which improve the health of agricultural migratory workers and their families.

"(e) The Secretary may enter into contracts with public and private entities to—

"(1) assist the States in the implementation and enforcement of acceptable environmental health standards, including enforcement of standards for sanitation in migrant labor camps and applicable Federal and State pesticide control standards; and

"(2) conduct projects and studies to assist the several States in the assessment of problems related to camp and field sanitation, pesticide hazards, and other environmental health problems faced by agricultural migratory workers.

"(f) (1) For payments under grants and contracts under this section, there are authorized to be appropriated $50,000,000 for the fiscal year ending June 30, 1975; and $55,000,000 for the fiscal year ending June 30, 1976.

"(2) Of the funds appropriated under paragraph (1) of this subsection for any fiscal year, not more than 30 per centum of such funds shall be used for grants and contracts under subsection (d) for the fiscal year ending June 30, 1975, and not more than 20 per centum of such funds shall be used for such grants and contracts for any succeeding fiscal year. Of the funds appropriated under this subsection for any fiscal year, not more than 10 per centum of such funds shall be used for contracts under subsection (e).

"(g) No grant may be made or contract entered into under this section unless an application therefor has been submitted to and approved by the Secretary. Such application shall be submitted in such form and manner and shall contain such information as the Secretary shall prescribe. The Secretary may not approve an application for a grant under subsection (c) for a migrant health center unless he determines that—

"(1) the center will compile and report such statistics and other information as the Secretary may require with respect to (A) the cost of its operations, (B) the patterns of use of its services, (C) the availability, accessibility, and acceptability of its services, and (D) such other matters as the Secretary may require;

"(2) the center will demonstrate its financial responsibility by the use of accounting procedures and other requirements as may be prescribed by the Secretary in order to insure that the center will maintain a solvent operation;

"(3) the center (A) has or will have a contractual or other arrangement with the agency of the State in which it provides services, which administers or supervises the administration of a State plan approved under title XIX of the Social Security Act, for the payment of all or a part of the center's costs in providing health services to persons who are eligible for medical assistance under such a State plan, or (B) has made or will make every reasonable effort to enter into such an arrangement; and

"(4) the center has made or will make and will continue to make every reasonable effort to collect appropriate reimbursement for its costs in providing health services to persons who are entitled to insurance benefits under title XVIII of such Act, to medical assistance under a State plan approved under title XIX of such Act, or to assistance for medical expenses under any other public assistance program or private health insurance program.

"(h) Contracts under this section may be entered into without regard to sections 3648 and 3709 of the Revised Statutes (31 U.S.C. 529; 42 U.S.C. 5)."

Sec. 402. (a) The Secretary of Health, Education, and Welfare (hereinafter in this section referred to as the "Secretary") shall conduct or arrange for the conduct of a study of—

(1) the quality of housing which is available to agricultural migratory workers in the United States during the period of their employment in seasonal agricultural activities while away from their permanent abodes;

(2) the effect on the health of such workers of deficiencies in their housing conditions during such period; and

(3) Federal, State, and local government standards respecting housing conditions for such workers during such period and the adequacy of the enforcement of such standards.

In conducting or arranging for the conduct of such study, the Secretary shall consult with the Secretary of Housing and Urban Development.

(b) Such study shall be completed and a report detailing the findings of the study and the recommendations of the Secretary for Federal action (including legislation) respecting such housing conditions shall be submitted to the Committee on Interstate and Foreign Commerce of the House of Representatives and the Committee on Labor and Public Welfare of the Senate within eighteen months of the date of the enactment of the first Act making appropriations for such study.

Notes

NOTES TO CHAPTER 1
THE PROBLEM OF MIGRANT HEALTH

1. The situation of migrant workers in America today is most recently and extensively considered in two sets of hearings before the Subcommittee on Migratory Labor of the Committee on Labor and Public Welfare, United States Senate. Under subcommittee chairman Walter F. Mondale, the ninety-first Congress first and second sessions held sixteen days of hearings on the general subject of "Migrant and Seasonal Farmworker Powerlessness," from June 9, 1969 sporatically through July 24, 1970. These hearings are published by the Government Printing Office, Washington, D.C. 1970 for Part 1 through Part 8-A, 1971 for Parts 8-B and 8-C. Under subcommittee chairman Adlai E. Stevenson, III, the ninety-second Congress first and second sessions held nine days of hearings on the general subject of "Farmworkers in Rural America, 1971–1972," from July 22, 1971 sporatically through June 20, 1972. These hearings with an appendix are published by the Government Printing Office, Washington, D.C., 1972 for Part 1 through Part 5-B.

   For the causes of the need for migratory labor, see Paul S. Taylor, "Origins and Growth of Migratory Seasonal Labor in Agriculture," Farmworkers in Rural America, 1971–1972, Part 5-B, pp. 3892–916.
2. Peter Barnes, "The Great American Land Grab," The New Republic, June 5, 1971 pp. 19–23. Reprinted in "Farmworkers in Rural America, 1971–1972" Part 1, pp. 133–7.
3. Ibid.
4. Philip Moore, testifying before the Senate Subcommittee on Migratory Labor, July 21, 1970. "Migrant and Seasonal Farmworker Powerlessness, Part 8-B," pages 5499–521.

   A.V. Krebs, Jr., "Montgomery Street: How it Controls California

Agriculture—The Second Gold Rush." San Francisco Magazine 12 (February 1970). Reprinted in "Farmworkers in Rural America, 1971–1972, Part 3-A," pp. 742–5.

"A Profile of California Agribusiness," Agribusiness Accountability Project, Washington, D.C., January 1972. Reprinted in "Farmworkers in Rural America, 1971–1972, Part 5-A," pp. 3055–136.

5. Angus McDonald, "The Family Farm is the Most Efficient Unit of Agricultural Production," "Farmworkers in Rural America, 1971–1972, Part 3C," pp. 2067–2073.

J. Patrick Madden, "Economies of Size in Farming—Theory, Analytical Procedures, and a Review of Selected Studies," (Economic Research Service, United States Department of Agriculture, Agricultural Report No. 107, Washington, D.C.: Government Printing Office, 1967). Reprinted in "Farmworkers in Rural American, 1971–1972, Part 5A," pp. 3467–554.

Michael Perelman, "Efficiency and Agriculture," "Farmworkers in Rural America, 1971–1972, Part 5B" pp. 3869–91.

6. John Steinbeck, *The Grapes of Wrath* (New York, Viking Press, 1939). Carey McWilliams, *Factories in the Field* (Boston, Little, Brown and Company, 1939). Carey McWilliams, *Ill Fares the Land* (New York, Barnes & Noble, 1967).

7. "Migrant Health Insurance Feasibility Study, Volume III, Family Survey," Control Systems Research, Incorporated, Arlington, Va. Submitted under contract to Office of Economic Opportunity, Washington, D.C., February 28, 1971, pp. 2–3. Hereinafter referred to as CSR-III.

8. "The Hired Farm Working Force of 1971," Rural Manpower Developments, Rural Manpower Service, U.S. Department of Labor, October 1972. Hereinafter referred to as DOL, 1972.

9. "Migrant Health Insurance Feasibility Study, Volume I, Rationale for a Health Insurance Demonstration," Control Systems Research, Incorporated, Arlington, Va. Submitted under contract to Office of Economic Opportunity, Washington, D.C., February 28, 1971, pp. 16, 19–21. Hereinafter referred to as CSR I.

10. "The Migratory Farm Labor Problem in the United States," 1969 Report of the Committee on Labor and Public Welfare, United States Senate, Subcommittee on Migratory Labor. (Washington, D.C.: U.S. Government Printing Office, 1969), pp. 4–5. Hereinafter referred to as 1969 Senate Report.

11. CSR-I, p. 10.

12. CSR-I, pp. 3, 8.

13. CSR-III, pp. 18–19.

14. 1969 Senate Report, pp. 6–7.

15. "Evaluation, Design and Analysis of Migrant Health Delivery Systems," Community Change, Incorporated, Sausalito, California. Submitted under contract to U.S. Department of Health, Education, and Welfare, Washington, D.C., July 15, 1971, p. 53. Hereinafter referred to as CCI.

16. 1969 Senate Report, p. 11.
17. DOL, 1972.
18. "The Hired Farm Working Force of 1972." Agricultural Economic Report No. 239, Economic Research Service, U.S. Department of Agriculture, Washington, D.C.
19. CSR-III, p. 16.
20. 1969 Senate Report, p. 34.
21. Testimony of Migrant Research Project before Senate Subcommittee on Migratory Labor, April 15, 1970. Printed in "Migrant and Seasonal Farmworker Powerlessness, Part 7-B" pp. 4827–28.
22. These well documented points are graphically illustrated in A. Donabedian, S.J. Axelrod, C. Swearingen, and J. Jameson, *Medical Care Chart Book, Fifth Edition* (Ann Arbor, Michigan: University of Michigan Bureau of Public Health Economics, 1972). See also Ronald Andersen, Rachel McL. Greeley, Joanna Kravits, and Odin W. Anderson, *Health Service Use: National Trends and Variations,* (DHEW Publications No. (HSM) 73–3004, Rockville, Maryland: U.S. Government Printing Office, 1972).
23. Robert Gnaizda, testifying before the Senate Subcommittee on Migratory Labor, April 15, 1970. "Migrant and Seasonal Farmworker Powerlessness, Part 7-B," p. 4697.
24. H. Peter Chase, N. Noreen Welch, Stephen Barnett, Franklin Briese, and Michael L. Krassner, "Pesticides and U.S. Farm Labor Families," unpublished manuscript from University of Colorado Medical Center, Denver, and Colorado Rural Legal Services, Boulder, Colorado.
25. Paul Monahan and Victor Eisner (eds.), *California Migrant Health Physician Symposium, May, 1968* (Berkeley; California State Department of Public Health, undated) pp. B6–B8.
26. H. Peter Chase, Vijay Kumar, Janice H. Dodds, Howard E. Sauberlich, Robert M. Hunter, Robert S. Burton, and Vaughn Spaulding, "Nutritional Status of Preschool Mexican-American Migrant Farm Children," *American Journal of Diseases of Children* 122 (October 1971): 316–24.
27. Gus Alevizos, Robert J. Walsh and Phil Aherne (compilers and editors), *Socioeconomic Issues of Health* (Chicago, American Medical Association, 1973), p. 27.
28. Graciela Delgado, C.L. Brumback, Mary Brice Deaver, "Eating Patterns Among Migrant Families," *Public Health Reports* 76 (April 1961): 349–55.
29. V.F. Thiele, M. Brin, M.V. Dibble, "Preliminary Biochemical Findings in Negro Migrant Workers at King Ferry, New York," *American Journal of Clinical Nutrition* 21 (November 1968): 1229–38.
30. Ibid., p. 1236.
31. Ibid., p. 1238.
32. The Field Foundation findings are printed as testimony to the Senate Subcommittee on Migratory Labor in "Migrant and Seasonal

Farmworker Powerlessness, Part 8-A" (Washington, D.C.: Government Printing Office, 1970). The testimony was given on July 20, 1970.

33. Robert Coles, in 1969 Senate Report, pp. 17–18.
34. CSR-I, pp. 25–33.
35. Ibid., pp. 12–15.
36. A large portion of the information for this and the following section comes from "Federal and State Statutes Relating to Farmworkers, A Compilation" prepared for the Senate Subcommittee on Migratory Labor (Washington, D.C.: Government Printing Office, 1972).
37. Ibid., p. 177.
37a. Ronald B. Taylor, *Sweatshops in the Sun: Child Labor on the Farm* (Boston: Beacon Press, 1973).
38. Gnaizda, op. cit., pp. 4590ff. The Department of Labor itself confirmed Gnaizda's findings in its own study under Secretary James D. Hodgson.
39. Raymond C. Lerner, "Social Factors in Medical Care: A Study of Migrant Health Problems," unpublished manuscript, Columbia University School of Public Health, January 1964.
40. Ibid., p. 50.
41. Ibid., p. 53.
42. Ibid., p. 107.
43. Ibid., p. 110.
44. 1969 Senate Report, p. 31.
45. CSR-III, pp. 6–7.
46. Alfonzo J. Gonzalez, "Brief Analysis of H.R. 7597: The Farm Labor Contractor Registration Act Amendments of 1973," *Clearinghouse Review*, January 1974, pp. 537–38.
47. Margaret Greenfield, "County Residence Rules as a Deterrent to Medical Care of Migrant Workers," Institute of Governmental Studies, University of California, Berkeley (February, 1964), unpublished.
48. C.N. Theodore and G.E. Sutter, "Distribution of Physicians, Hospitals, and Hospital Beds in the U.S. by Census Region, State, County and Metropolitan Area," (Chicago: American Medical Association, 1966)
49. Milton I. Roemer and Daniel M. Anzel, "Health Needs and Services of the Rural Poor," *Medical Care Review* 25 (May and June, 1968) p. 380.
50. Rashi Fein, *The Doctor Shortage: An Economic Diagnosis* (Washington, D.C., Brookings, 1967), pp. 90ff.
51. Milton I. Roemer and William Shonick, "HMO Performance: The Recent Evidence," *Milbank Memorial Fund Quarterly: Health and Society* 51 (summer 1973), p. 301.
52. Roemer and Anzel, "Health Needs and Services."
53. Ibid., p. 479.
54. Donald L. Madison, "Unsolicited Proposal to the National Health Service Corps for a Program of Evaluative Research in Connection with Assignments of Physicians and Dentists in Rural Communities," April 14, 1972, pp. 2–3.

55. Roemer and Anzel, "Health Needs and Services," pp. 480ff.
56. CSR-III, pp. 33, 63, 67.
57. Chase, Kumar, Dodds, Sauberlich, Hunter, Burton, Spaulding, "Nutritional Status of Preschool Mexican-American Migrant Farm Children," in "Migrant and Seasonal Farmworker Powerlessness, Part 8-A" Hearings before the Senate Subcommittee on Migratory Labor, July 20, 1970, pp. 5135–43.
58. CCI, p. 55.
59. Gnaizda, op. cit.
60. Chase et al., supra note 57.
61. 1969 Senate Report, p. 18.
62. Monahan and Eisner (eds.), op. cit., p. B2.
63. Roy Penchansky and Daniel Fox, "Frequency of Referral and Patient Characteristics in Group Practice," *Medical Care* 8 (September–October 1970): 368.
64. Barbara Starfield, "Health Services Research: A Working Model," *New England Journal of Medicine* 289 (July 19, 1973): 132–6.
65. A. Donabedian, *Guide to Medical Care Administration*, Volume II. New York, American Public Health Association, 1969.
66. J. Richard Udry and Naomi M. Morris, "A Spoonful of Sugar Helps the Medicine Go Down," *American Journal of Public Health* 61 (April 1971).
67. Barry Blackwell, "Patient Compliance," *New England Journal of Medicine* 289 (1973): 249–52.

NOTES TO CHAPTER 2
THE CLASSICAL MIGRANT HEALTH PROGRAM

1. "Evaluation, Design and Analysis of Migrant Health Delivery Systems," Community Change, Incorporated, Sausalito, California. Submitted under contract to U.S. Department of Health, Education, and Welfare, Washington, D.C., July 15, 1971, p. 26. Hereinafter referred to as CCI.
2. "Evaluatory Study on Operations of the Migrant Health Program under the Migrant Health Act," New York, American Public Health Association, December 30, 1964, Unpublished report. Hereinafter called APHA.
3. CCI, p. 26.
4. "Health for the Harvesters. Decade of Hope, 1960–1970," Berkeley, California State Department of Public Health, p. 26.
5. Robert Gnaizda, testifying before the Senate Subcommittee on Migratory Labor, April 15, 1970. "Migrant and Seasonal Farmworker Powerlessness, Part 7-B," p. 4589 ff.
6. CCI, pp. 27–8.

7. Oliver M. Korshin, "Site visit—Maricopa County Migrant Health Project, Phoenix, Arizona, April 30, 1969," memorandum to the files, Public Health Service Region IX, May 6, 1969.
8. APHA, p. 22.

NOTES TO CHAPTER 3 PROPOSED ALTERNATIVES TO THE "CLASSICAL" SOLUTION

1. "The Migratory Farm Labor Problem in the United States," 1969 Report of the Committee on Labor and Public Welfare, United States Senate, Subcommittee on Migratory Labor (Washington, D.C.: U.S. Government Printing Office, 1969).
2. H. Peter Chase, Vijay Kumar, Janice H. Dodds, Howard E. Sauberlich, Robert M. Hunter, Robert S. Burton, and Vaughn Spaulding, "Nutritional Status of Preschool Mexican-American Migrant Farm Children," *American Journal of Diseases of Children* 122 (October 1971): 316–24.
3. John E. Kleinert, "Migrant Children in Florida, Phase II Report," University of Miami, Florida Migratory Child Survey Center, 1969. Kleinert found that 3% of the adult migrants he questioned had experienced what they regarded as a need for medical care, nearly 8% a need for medicines, about 11% medical care for their children, and 11% medicines for their children.
4. "Migrant Health Insurance Feasibility Study, 3 volumes," Control Systems Research, Inc., Arlington, Va. Submitted under contract to Office of Economic Opportunity, Washington, D.C., February 28, 1971. Hereinafter referred to as CSR-I (volume 1) CSR-II (volume 2) and CSR-III (volume 3).
5. CSR-I, pp. 36–37.
6. CSR-I, pp. 46–47.
7. CSR-I, p. 71.
8. CSR-I, p. 68.
9. CSR-I, p. 69.
10. Milton I. Roemer, private communication, 1971.
11. CSR-III, pp. 8–9.
12. Maurice King, *Medical Care in Developing Countries* (London: Oxford Univer-Press, 1966), p. 2:10.
13. Thomas Bodenheimer, "Mobile Units: A Solution to Rural Health Problems?" *Medical Care* 7 (March–April 1969): 144–54.
14. Ibid., p. 144.
15. Herbert A. Simon, *Administrative Behavior*, second edition (New York: The Macmillan Company, 1957).

NOTES TO CHAPTER 4
ADMINISTRATIVE CONSIDERATIONS

1. Anthony Downs, *Inside Bureaucracy* (Boston: Little, Brown, 1967).
2. Harold Seidman, *Politics, Position, and Power: The Dynamics of Federal Organization* (New York: Oxford University Press, 1970), p. 107.
3. Report of the Secretary's Committee to Study the Public Health Service Commissioned Corps, Dr. John A. Perkins, Chairman. Washington, D.C.: U.S. Department of Health, Education, and Welfare, June 21, 1971.
4. See James D. Thompson, *Organizations in Action* (New York: McGraw-Hill, 1967), especially chapter 2, and Seidman, *Politics, Position, and Power: The Dynamics of Federal Organization,* pp. 122ff.
5. CCI.
6. Downs, *Inside Bureaucracy.*
7. Ibid., p. 111.
8. The story of this young osteopath was recounted in the National Affairs section of Newsweek, July 27, 1970, page 21.

NOTES TO CHAPTER 5
THE POLITICS OF MIGRANT HEALTH

1. House of Representatives, Report N. 2253, "Health Clinics for Domestic Migratory Farmworkers," August 20, 1962, p. 3.
2. Ibid., p. 3.
3. Ibid., p. 6.
4. For an interesting sketch of Rogers' attitude in a legislative situation, see Eric Redman's *The Dance of Legislation* (New York: Simon and Schuster, 1973), pp. 89ff.
5. Beverlee A. Myers, "Health Maintenance Organizations: Objectives and Issues," Rockville, Md.: Health Services and Mental Health Administration, 1971.
6. Ibid.
7. Jerome L. Schwartz, *Medical Plans and Health Care: Consumer Participation in Policy Making with a Special Section on Medicare* (Springfield, Ill.: Charles C. Thomas, 1968).

Index

About the Author

Budd Shenkin, a native of Philadelphia, Pennsylvania, majored in history and graduated with honors from Harvard College, received his M.D. degree from Harvard Medical School, and interned in pediatrics at the University of California in San Francisco. He then joined the Community Health Service of the U.S. Public Health Service in Washington, D.C., where for two years he helped administer the national Migrant Health Program.

Following this he was awarded a three year fellowship from the PHS. During these years he received a master's degree from the Graduate School of Public Policy at the University of California, Berkeley, did research on the Swedish medical care system at the Stockholm School of Economics, and was a post-doctoral fellow at Yale, writing professional articles on Swedish medical care and articles advocating giving patients their medical records. He also consulted with the United States Congress on the Migrant Health Program. After spending another year with the office of the Assistant Secretary for Health and the Bureau of Health Services Research in Washington, he returned to California where he now lives in Berkeley with his wife and two sons, and teaches at the University of California at San Francisco.